VACCINES

VACCINES

A Reappraisal

RICHARD MOSKOWITZ, MD

Foreword by Mary Holland, JD

Skyhorse Publishing

Skyhorse Publishing books may be purchased in bulk at special discounts for sales promotion, corporate gifts, fund-raising, or educational purposes. Special editions can also be created to specifications. For details, contact the Special Sales Department, Skyhorse Publishing, 307 West 36th Street, 11th Floor, New York, NY 10018 or info@skyhorsepublishing.com.

Skyhorse® and Skyhorse Publishing® are registered trademarks of Skyhorse Publishing, Inc.®, a Delaware corporation.

Visit our website at www.skyhorsepublishing.com.

10 9 8 7 6 5 4 3

Library of Congress Cataloging-in-Publication Data is available on file.

Cover design by Rain Saukas
Cover photograph: iStockphoto

Print ISBN: 978-1-5107-2256-9
Ebook ISBN: 978-1-5107-2258-3

Printed in the United States of America

DEDICATION

To the pursuit of real science, conducted in an objective and disinterested manner, rather than simply to sell a product, or advertise conclusions already determined in advance, as described by the late Richard Feynman, professor of Theoretical Physics at Caltech and winner of the Nobel Prize for Physics in 1965:

> Science creates a power through its knowledge, a power to do things. It does not give instructions as to how to use it for good rather than evil. Scientists' statements are approximate, never absolutely certain. We must leave room for doubt, or there is no progress and no learning. There is no learning without having to pose a question, and a question requires doubt. Before you begin an experiment, you must not know the answer. If you already know the answer, there is no need to gather any evidence; and to judge the evidence, you must take all of it, not just the parts you like. That's a responsibility that scientists feel toward each other, a kind of morality.
>
> Science has had long experience with ignorance, doubt, and uncertainty. Our freedom to doubt was born of a struggle against authority, a very deep and powerful struggle. Permit us to question, to doubt, to not be sure: that's all we ask. We must not forget the importance of this struggle, or we may lose what we have gained. Here lies a responsibility to society, to pass on what we have learned, and to leave future scientists a free hand. We make a grave error if we say we have the answers now, suppressing all discussion and criticism, and thus doom mankind to be chained to authority, to the limits of our present understanding, as has been done so often before!
>
> —*The Pleasure of Finding Things Out*

CONTENTS

FOREWORD

All over the world, governments, medical institutions, and manufacturers are trying to persuade or compel people to vaccinate themselves and their children from cradle to grave. The modern world prizes vaccines as the signal triumph of medicine over disease, its quintessential achievement.

But does this paradigm make sense? Should we accept it? Should we permit governments to go beyond recommending vaccines for infants to mandating them for everyone? Is the science "settled" as firmly and beyond doubt as we have been led to believe? In his *Vaccines: A Reappraisal,* Richard Moskowitz, MD, asks these questions in a systematic way, and provides critical thinking and careful scholarship to help us try to answer them, as well as highlighting important scientific work that has been and still remains to be done.

Dr. Moskowitz is a practicing physician with fifty years of experience, and the book he offers is clearly written and easily accessible for readers with or without a medical background. In addition to lessons drawn from his own practice and that of like-minded colleagues, it provides an extensive review of

1. official pronouncements from industry and various government agencies;
2. epidemiological and basic-science research from the scientific literature;
3. tragic stories of real people and damaged lives; and
4. news stories bearing on all of the above.

There are many books critical of vaccines on the market today. What is unique about this one is its comprehensive analysis of the subject as a whole, from the much-loved but sadly vanishing perspective of an old-time family doctor.

Dr. Moskowitz sees our present vaccine policy as a vast, costly, and dangerous experiment that is out of control, obscenely profitable, and badly in need of independent regulation. He catalogues the risks of each individual vaccine, as well as those of the vaccination process *per se.* He explains how the industry's in-house safety trials, and the government's Vaccine Adverse Event Reporting System (VAERS) and National Vaccine Injury Compensation Program (VICP), systematically ignore and underreport important classes of injuries caused by vaccines, so that the true extent of their burden on the medical system remains hidden and to that extent unknowable.

As a kind of bottom line, he emphasizes the basic right of every patient to free and informed consent, which dovetails closely with my own work as a human rights lawyer, and undoubtedly explains why he sought me out to write this foreword. To put vaccines in their proper place, he advocates nothing more radical than simply holding them to the same standards that all other prescription drugs must abide by, namely,

1. honoring every individual's right to refuse them;
2. requiring them to undergo the same degree of rigorous testing;
3. providing complete information about their adverse effects;
4. extending the definition of these beyond the incredibly narrow restrictions in use today; and
5. restoring the legal liability of manufacturers for damages caused by vaccines that remains in force for every other drug.

Like my own, Dr. Moskowitz's opposition to mandatory vaccination adheres closely to the letter and the spirit of the 2005 Universal Declaration on Bioethics and Human Rights, which affirms that, apart from a public health emergency, the interests of science and society must not be allowed to override the right of all people to make medical decisions for themselves and their children.

Our current vaccine policy shockingly deviates from that fundamental principle, which a traumatized world adopted as a result of the atrocious crimes against humanity committed in World War II. Both the Nuremburg Code of 1945 and the 2005 Universal Declaration that supplemented it were signed by more than 190 countries, including the United States, and have established unequivocally that medical care must not be subject to governmental coercion, except in the rarest and most extreme circumstances.

In 2015, a small measles outbreak among visitors to Disneyland prompted the state of California to enact a law prohibiting infants and children from attending any school or preschool, whether public or private, unless they are fully compliant with the state's vaccine mandates, a draconian measure that abandons sensible public health practice as well as basic human rights. Since then, many other states and even the federal government are considering similar laws, merely because a small but growing minority of parents are continuing to question and refuse some vaccines for their children.

Passionately committed to safeguarding these rights, Dr. Moskowitz points out that by transgressing this core principle of medical ethics and international law, coercive mandates also erode the mutual trust that the doctor-patient relationship and ultimately the art and science of medicine are built upon.

As it happens, a sizable number of developed countries in Europe, North America, and Asia that have relaxed such mandates have not only escaped any major health problems as a result, but have recorded consistently lower infant mortality rates and scored better on other standard health measures as well, without cruelly forcing parents to choose between educating their children and refusing to vaccinate them.

The acrimonious public dialogue about vaccines will probably continue, and could become even more polarizing in the months to come. But this book provides invaluable help for parents seeking another perspective before making up their minds: it is well thought out and filled with scientific insight, common sense, and practical wisdom.

—Mary Holland, JD, research scholar, NYU School of Law

INTRODUCTION

The practice of vaccinating children to prevent infectious diseases, especially those that are nonthreatening or already in decline, has long been and still remains deeply troubling to me, because of perceived logical inconsistencies in the concept and deep misgivings about their safety as a result of them. Along with a great deal of reading and thinking about vaccines, fifty years of clinical experience treating children and adults have amply validated these concerns and added several new ones.

As more and more vaccines continue to be developed and mandated without regulation or restraint, often for no more compelling reason than that we possess the technical capacity to make them, the parents whose children are about to be injected deserve an explanation that will address their doubts and fears in a sympathetic, respectful, and thoughtfully reasoned manner.

Needless to say, I am well aware that even questioning these mandates has placed me beyond the pale of what most people sincerely and devoutly believe, backed up by the full weight of opinion from established authorities such as the CDC, the American Academy of Pediatrics, and the vast preponderance of the medical community as a whole.

Indeed, these same intelligent and literate people who believe in science and value mandatory vaccinations are an important part of the audience for whom this book is intended. I'm thinking of all the parents who conscientiously vaccinate their kids with little hesitation or soul-searching, and of all the doctors and scientists who are deeply committed to the scientific worldview, as I am, and perhaps roll their eyes at my presuming to question the wisdom of a procedure that has won broad acclaim across the scientific world as one of the best that modern medicine has to offer.

The ever-increasing number of parents who honestly believe that their children were killed or maimed by vaccines and must live with that existential reality every day of their lives hardly need my arguments to convince them. It is that far greater multitude of scientists, doctors, and parents who gladly or reluctantly vaccinate their kids and perhaps resent those whose children are getting off scot-free, seemingly at their expense, whom I would also like to reason with; and I would be foolish indeed to imagine that my task will be an easy one.

Even if we could be sure that vaccines were harmless, the fact remains that our country requires all children to receive them, and indeed more of them than anywhere else in the world, without adequate safety studies, due regard for basic differences in individual susceptibility, or the values and wishes of the parents and the children themselves.

In a functioning democracy, most people can accept the reality that laws may be necessary for the public good that they dislike or even strongly disagree with. But what is at stake in this case is the routine injection of live viruses, foreign proteins, toxic chemical adjuvants, and a witches' brew of antibiotics, detergents, acid and alkaline buffers, hydrocarbons, a variety of animal cells, and foreign DNA and proteins directly into the bloodstream of entire populations, and especially of our newly born children at the earliest and most vulnerable stage of their development.

For that reason alone, the public is surely entitled to convincing proof, beyond any reasonable doubt, utilizing science of the highest quality, and readily understandable to the lay reader, that vaccination is a safe and effective procedure, in no way injurious to health, and that the threat of the corresponding natural diseases remains sufficiently compelling to warrant the mass vaccination of everyone, even against their will if necessary.

Unfortunately, such proofs have never been given, or even thought necessary; and even if routine mass vaccination could be shown to be uniformly safe and effective, the decision would remain in the end a moral and political one, involving issues of public health and safety far too important to be settled by any purely scientific or technical criteria, or indeed by *any* criteria less authoritative than the clearly articulated sense of the community about to be subjected to it.

For all of these reasons, I want to invite my readers to think very carefully about vaccines and our present policy regarding them, not least because the concerns of parents who decide not to vaccinate their children are so rarely acknowledged or taken seriously. For myself, as a family physician who has cared for many such children over the years, I cannot keep silent about the major epidemic of vaccine-related suffering and disability, sufficient to break any heart, that continues unabated, remains largely unacknowledged, and cries out at the very least for caution, restraint, and simple compassion for the viewpoint of those whose lived experience, whatever may have caused it, is so tragically different from that of everyone else privileged enough to be ignorant of or somehow unmoved by their loss.

In what follows, I make no claim to absolute truth or final answers. I am a family doctor, not a research scientist, and at bottom I am trying simply to make sense of my own clinical experience. What I offer is an ensemble of observed facts, clinical and basic scientific research, news reports from the media, actual cases from my practice, and such reflections and hypotheses as have occurred to me and other colleagues in the field to try to explain and integrate them. My aim is to provide an overview of the subject that will be accessible to a general literate audience, regardless of scientific training or background. I will feel well rewarded if my words, my reasoning, and the commingled sadness, fear, and outrage I have long felt about this subject will help to promote a healthy debate and to elicit more of the rigorous scientific work that still needs to be done.

I also write with a sense of urgency, because the time-honored rights of patients to refuse unwanted medical treatment and to make such decisions on behalf of their children are now being challenged as never before. I am not a teetotaler who rejects all vaccines under all circumstances. The essence of my position is simply that vaccines by their very nature have a major downside that has largely been ignored, so that it is reckless in the extreme to continue mandating them—and indeed more and more of them without limit or restraint—until these dangers are taken seriously, understood in a broader context, and assessed in a more careful and systematic fashion.

Under these circumstances, the risks of vaccination are compounded by the concerted efforts of the industry, the CDC, and the doctors who speak for them to keep them hidden, and the considerable shift in perspective that is needed to recognize them. In a sense, the risk of major complications that every vaccine carries with it is merely a special case of the risk that accompanies every other drug with sufficient chemical power to accomplish what we ask of it; but vaccines alone are required of every child, and their bad outcomes are not merely idiosyncratic aberrations, but are in fact built into their design, as I will presently show.

Likewise, although such misfortunes belong in the wastebasket category of "side effects" that eventually come to haunt every potent drug, the maker of other medicines that kill or harm can at least be held liable for damages in the worst cases; only the vaccine manufacturers are shielded by an Act of Congress and a 2011 Supreme Court ruling from having to assume even that minimal degree of responsibility for their most egregious faults and tragic miscalculations. By thus indulging an already rich and powerful industry on the grounds that vaccines are "unavoidably unsafe," and excluding any redress for all but a tiny minority of the helpless children who are nevertheless required to receive them, both we as citizens and the government that claims to represent us have abandoned the same basic principles of justice to which we nevertheless continue to profess our allegiance.

Given that the safety of these agents continues to be so polarizing, and the rationale for requiring them of everyone is based on a comprehensive, long-term strategy rather than a genuine public health emergency, the safest and wisest course would be simply to make them optional, offering them to those who want them, and allowing parents to exercise their moral and legal right to choose which treatments are appropriate for their children, and which diseases, if any, to vaccinate their children against.

Both the right to refuse medical treatment and the authority of parents to do so on behalf of their children have been recognized and enshrined in the laws of almost every state for more than a century; and even in the most liberal of them, the number of children actually claiming such a personal-belief exemption has never exceeded a tiny fraction of the population. Nevertheless, to a degree without precedent or parallel elsewhere, our uniquely American sanctification of vaccines as not only unquestionably safe and effective, but also a kind of magic wand against infectious diseases of every kind, has given a free ride and indeed a blank check to the giant multinationals who make them and the small coterie of physicians who advocate on their behalf.

What is new and different about the present moment is just that their long-cherished goal of vaccinating everyone without exception seems for the first time tantalizingly within reach, thanks to a small cluster of measles cases among travelers to Disneyland involving less than 150 in all, but including some dozens who became infected after the vacationers returned to their home states.

As if to forestall the logical conclusion that the measles vaccine isn't all that effective, the industry has cleverly repackaged this rapid and easy transmission of the virus across state lines from a minor and wholly typical outbreak into the looming and dreaded semblance of a major public health emergency. By fear-mongering in the media, lobbying state legislatures, and mounting lavish advertising campaigns in support of universal compliance with existing vaccine mandates, the powerful vaccine lobby has already succeeded in proposing new laws in more than half the states that would eliminate all personal-belief exemptions entirely.

The most comprehensive and draconian of these was recently signed into law in California, one of the bluest of the "blue" states, with a long and proud history of civil rights, democratic values, and a thriving alternative-medicine community, ominously trumped by what Governor Brown naïvely proclaimed as "clear scientific evidence" in the act of signing it. If it succeeds in withstanding the legal challenges that are already in progress, the only allowed exceptions remaining will be for established medical contraindications, which have always been notoriously few, defined ever more narrowly, applicable to only one vaccine at a time, and subject to review on a yearly basis.

I will leave aside for the moment the almost embarrassingly obvious illogic of this strategy, namely,

- that a hundred and fifty cases of the measles are so insignificant in the scheme of things;
- that it makes no sense to blame these outbreaks on the unvaccinated kids, since the majority of cases were actually vaccinated, as has been uniformly true of similar outbreaks in the past;
- that vaccination rates are already well over 90% in the United States for most vaccines, and over 95% in many locations where the measles have actually broken out, statistics that are and have always been among the highest in the world; and
- that it defies both epidemiological experience and ordinary common sense to imagine that even vaccinating everyone without exception, as the new laws require, would do much if anything to stop these small outbreaks that have continued to occur ever since the vaccines were introduced.

While I can certainly imagine that the right to refuse treatment and the authority of parents to decide for their children might need to be waived for a brief period in the event of a genuine public health emergency, that is most assuredly what such small clusters of ordinary childhood illnesses are not. This brings me to another obvious point: if vaccines were equal to the extravagant claims made for them, if they were truly effective in conferring a genuine immunity similar to that acquired by coming down with and recovering from the natural disease, then the unvaccinated kids would pose a danger only to themselves, based on a free choice of their own making.

It feels even more embarrassing to have to repeat what at bottom we all know, and what even the most zealous pro-vaccine advocates would have to admit, that vaccine-mediated immunity falls far short of that standard, being neither genuine, nor long-lasting, nor nearly as effective as we are being told, and that measles, mumps, chicken pox, and influenza, for example, are diseases that I, like virtually everyone of my generation, came down with as a child and recovered from without complications or sequelae.

In short, we all know or should know that vaccination is essentially an artifice, designed to trick the immune mechanism into providing a semblance or counterfeit of immunity that is partial, defective, and temporary at best, and that carries substantial additional risks of its own that are inherent in the process.

While the debate continues, as I very much hope that it will, the immediate issue before the public is to preserve the frail remnant of personal liberty embodied in these few remaining exemptions that most citizens in our democracy have long been rightly proud of, which the influential and well-funded pro-vaccine lobby has always been eager to take away. My fervent hope and heartfelt plea is that good common sense will prevail and the American people will be sufficiently aroused to not let that happen.

PART I

THE VACCINATION PROCESS

Chapter 1

IMMUNITY, TRUE AND FALSE

NATURAL IMMUNITY

To understand vaccines in a comprehensive way, it is necessary to begin with the formative experience of coming down with and recovering from acute infectious diseases, because the mighty and concerted response that it calls for involves the principal functions of the immune system, which vaccination is meant to replace, and which are thus easily lost sight of in the heat of the debate.

Once again, measles provides the perfect example, as the most highly contagious of the typical childhood diseases; its attack rate approaches 100%, which means that nearly everyone exposed to the virus for the first time will come down with the illness, exhibiting signs and symptoms so memorable and so easy to recognize that parents of my generation commonly made the diagnosis themselves before the doctor ever saw the patient.

With its marked affinity for the mucous membranes of the upper respiratory tract, the measles virus is dispersed through the air by the sneezing and coughing of infected droplets, and inhaled by susceptible persons in the vicinity. Throughout its long incubation period of 10 to 14 days, the virus multiplies silently, first in the tonsils, adenoids, and accessory lymphoid tissues of the nasopharynx, then in the regional lymph nodes of the head and neck, and finally in the spleen, liver, thymus, and bone marrow, the major organs of the immune system, while the patient continues to feel well and generally exhibits few or no symptoms of any kind.[1]

By the time symptoms appear, specific antibodies are already detectable in the blood, and the height of the symptomatology roughly coincides with the peak of the antibody response.[2] But the illness that we know as the measles is nothing less than the concerted effort of the entire immune system to expel the virus from the blood, an all-important task that requires an impressive array of collaborative mechanisms and cannot be achieved by any one or part of them in isolation.

One of the simplest to understand is inflammatory sensitization of the epithelial cells lining the nasal, oral, and pharyngeal cavities, which are the first to receive the virus and thus admirably equipped to get rid of it, once again by sneezing and coughing.[3] A second indispensable component is the signaling and activation of monocytes and macrophages, two types of wandering, phagocytic cells that routinely police the blood, blood vessel walls, and connective tissues, in order to detect, engulf, and digest invading viruses,[4] while other types of phagocytic white cells, the neutrophils, basophils, and eosinophils, are called upon in the case of bacterial infections and exposure to various allergens and toxic chemicals, respectively. The elimination of foreign viruses and bacteria is further expedited by the complement system, a diverse fraction of serum proteins, which attach to and fragment the invading organism, thus preparing it for digestion.[5]

At the same time, yet another specialized class of smaller proteins and peptides, the interferons, interleukins, and other cytokines, enable the phagocytes to signal, communicate with, and direct one another to the areas where they are needed, and further assist in their work.[6] Taken together, all of these mechanisms constitute the most basic or "cellular" level of immunity, which not only provides our first line of defense against foreign invaders, but also initiates, coordinates, and regulates the process as a whole.

More or less simultaneously, cloned subsets of lymphocytes and plasma cells from the thymus and bone marrow synthesize specific antibodies directed against each particular invader, which assist in its destruction and removal; collectively, this special function is known as "humoral immunity." The inventory of these antibodies includes *opsonins*, which instigate phagocytosis of the viruses or bacteria; *agglutinins,* which facilitate clumping or agglutination of them or their antigens; and *precipitins,* which render them insoluble.[7]

All of these subtypes are clearly designed to assist the cellular mechanisms in completing their all-important task of attacking, destroying, and ultimately removing foreign microorganisms and antigens from the blood. Then and only then comes what might be called the "frosting on the cake," namely, the encryption of a permanent memory of the infection in the genetic material of these immunocompetent cells, to help them recognize the virus and respond to it even more promptly and efficiently should they encounter it again in the future.[8]

For most already healthy people, the immunity conferred by this splendid and massive outpouring is absolute, lifelong, and profoundly health-giving in two important senses. First, it is *specific,* in the obvious sense that virtually everyone who recovers from the measles will never again be susceptible to it, no matter how many times they are reexposed to the virus, or how many epidemics of the disease may be raging all around them.[9] Less often talked about but at least equally important is the *nonspecific* immunity that results from having activated the whole army of immune mechanisms across the board, thus priming the system to respond acutely, vigorously, and in a concerted fashion to whatever other infections it may encounter in the future.

In both respects, the natural immunity acquired by coming down with and recovering from acute diseases like the measles, typically characterized by fever and resulting in expulsion of the offending virus or bacterium from the blood, represents an enormous net gain for the general health of individuals and their descendants, and thereby also of the community, the nation, and ultimately of human life on the planet as a whole.

Amid the impressive array of new vaccines and the noisy bullying employed to promote them, it is easily forgotten that the growth, development, and maturation of a healthy immune system is accomplished mainly by learning how to mount such acute, vigorous responses to infection, and that the challenges of coming down with and recovering from illnesses of this type are the formative experiences by which this fundamental prerequisite of good health is achieved and maintained throughout life.

This basic truth is reinforced by a considerable body of epidemiological research to the effect that contracting and recovering from measles, mumps, chicken pox, influenza, and other acute childhood illnesses with fever provides significant protection against many chronic diseases later in life, including many autoimmune diseases and even cancer of various types.

In one such study, British scientists took careful histories from 300 women diagnosed with ovarian cancer, 300 women living in the same neighborhood, and another 300 women hospitalized for other gynecological conditions, and found that the incidence of ovarian cancer was significantly lower in women with a history of having contracted measles, mumps, rubella, or chicken pox in childhood, by 53%, 39%, 38%, and 34%, respectively.[10]

Another team comparing 603 European and Israeli melanoma patients with 627 matched population controls found that those who had experienced influenza, pneumonia, and indeed almost any febrile infection earlier in life were significantly less likely to develop melanoma than those who had not, roughly in proportion to the number of infections they reported.[11]

Similarly, 381 adults with glioma, a common type of brain tumor, were compared with 414 gender-, age-, and ethnicity-matched controls, with the result that the glioma patients were significantly less likely to have contracted chicken pox, or to show antibodies to the virus in their serum as evidence of it.[12]

An impressive array of studies document the same kind of inverse relationship between the incidence of leukemia and lymphoma and the number of febrile infections acquired earlier in life. Another study comparing 379 patients with cancer of many types and the same number of matched controls found that adults with a history of having acquired measles, mumps, rubella, chicken pox, pertussis, or scarlet fever were 20% less likely to develop genital, prostate, GI, skin, lung, or ENT cancer if they had experienced any one of these infections, 60% less likely if they experienced three or four of them, and 76% less likely if they experienced more than four.[13]

In addition, a considerable volume of research has documented still other health benefits accruing to adults who acquired the measles, mumps, chicken pox, and influenza naturally in childhood, rather than being vaccinated against them, namely, a significantly lower incidence of asthma, allergies, seizures, and a variety of autoimmune disorders,[14] including type 1 or insulin-dependent diabetes mellitus (IDDM), idiopathic thrombocytopenic purpura (ITP), Crohn's disease, ulcerative colitis, and even coronary artery disease later in life.[15]

The evolution of the measles through historical time teaches an even broader dimension of the same lesson. As vaccine advocates never tire of reminding us, measles was once a killer disease, and still carries a fatality rate of roughly 20% in populations encountering it for the first time;[16] it remains a major cause of death in many parts of Africa, where endemic malnutrition has kept that threat alive through generations of Western imperialism, the civil wars that have followed in its wake, and malnutrition, poverty, and the lack of any public health infrastructure to speak of.

Along with smallpox, it likewise became a powerful weapon for Cortez, Pizarro, and their *conquistadores* when they brought it with them to the New World,[17] and for Lord Jeffrey Amherst and other pioneer settlers of the American colonies and the future United States, who rarely scrupled about depopulating the native tribes they encountered by trading infected blankets along with muskets and powder for beaver pelts, tobacco, and the like.[18]

Yet within a few centuries of its appearance in Western Europe and the Americas, measles had evolved into a normal disease of childhood. The resulting "herd immunity" that protects susceptible people from minor exposures was sufficiently widespread before the first measles vaccine appeared in 1964 that, in spite of a prevalence of 400,000–800,000 cases annually in the United States,[19] almost all schoolchildren eventually acquired and recovered from it completely, without complications or sequelae; it nevertheless remained a major illness, with some risk of more serious complications like deafness, pneumonia, and encephalitis, and even death or brain damage in rare cases.

By the time I came down with the disease in the second grade, nonspecific mechanisms similar to the ones I have been describing were already in place, enabling me and my classmates to ride it out in bed with a high fever, florid rash, and lots of coughing and sneezing, meriting a home visit from our family doctor and a week off from school. In my own case, snugly ensconced under a tent with a vaporizer and plenty of TLC from my mother, who like many middle-class housewives of that happier era could afford to stay home and nurse me through it, I was lucky enough to remember my experience with the disease quite fondly on the whole.

But the main thing to be said about it is that it was in effect a graduation ceremony for my immune system, which was then and has since remained in a state of alert preparedness for any other infectious diseases that might come my way in later life, an experience to which I credit no small measure of the good health I still enjoy today.

Lurking in the shadows of the current vaccine debates is a vast cultural amnesia for this history, tempered by a vague nostalgia in many of the parents I see today for their grandparents' generations, when kids could still grow up and become healthy in the process of acquiring ordinary febrile infections like measles, mumps, and chicken pox.

For nursing mothers, another important tangible benefit of having recovered from measles and other such diseases is the presence of specific antibodies in their breast milk, which reliably transmits an acquired passive immunity to their babies at a time of life when their still undeveloped immune systems would be most vulnerable to these viruses, thus postponing their exposure to an age when they have already learned how to mount fever and other acute responses to minor infections as infants.[20]

In the case of the measles, it has also been the consensus of public health workers that large-scale outbreaks will no longer occur if 80% of the local population has come down with and recovered from the disease,[21] a "herd immunity" that works largely by protecting susceptible people from minor exposures. This statistic stands in marked contrast to the present situation, where the alleged herd immunity conferred by vaccination rates of 95% or more still fails to stop such outbreaks, thus further contributing to the widespread illusion of looming or imminent threats to the public health.

ARTIFICIAL OR VACCINE-MEDIATED IMMUNITY

All these benefits of natural immunity should be kept clearly in mind when discussing vaccines, because whatever good the latter accomplish inevitably falls far short of these goals. When a vaccine is ingested orally or injected into the blood, there is at most a brief inflammatory reaction at the portal of entry, but no local sensitization, no incubation period, no massive outpouring of lymphocytes, macrophages, and other phagocytes, no overt acute illness, and thus, above all, no obvious mechanism or pathway for getting rid of it.

After 14 days or so, yes, there are likely to be measurable titers of specific antibodies; and yes, the recipients of many, though not all, vaccines will be somewhat less likely to come down with the corresponding acute disease, at least in the near future, than they were before. But without the acute illness, there is no priming of the immune system as a whole, no significant improvement in the general health of the recipients or their neighbors, and no reliable mechanism for expelling the invading virus or bacterium; and where the latter actually *goes*, how it persuades the immune system to continue producing antibodies against it for years or even decades, as it is meant to do, and what price we have to pay for the partial, counterfeit immunity that they represent, are questions that it seems we are not supposed to ask, and can expect anything from haughty contempt to righteous indignation when we do.

What has always bothered me about vaccination is that it amounts to a conjuror's trick, designed to accomplish by deception precisely what the whole immune mechanism has seemingly evolved to prevent, namely, granting bacteria, viruses, and other foreign antigens free and immediate access to the bone marrow, spleen, liver, intestines, thymus, blood, and lymph nodes (i.e., the major internal organs of the immune system), with no reliable means of getting rid of them.

What continues to haunt me is what seems to me the logical conclusion that the continuous production of specific antibodies over the lifetime of the recipient, without the corresponding acute disease that they were designed to help get rid of, entails the ongoing physical presence of these vaccine organisms, or of highly antigenic substances produced by or from them, remaining in the body on a chronic and indeed more or less permanent basis.

Precisely how this persistent carrier state is accomplished is a mystery that for some reason is rarely discussed; but whatever the mechanism, it would seem to provide both a perfect recipe and all the necessary ingredients for eliciting autoimmune phenomena routinely and repeatedly throughout the lifetime of the recipients, whether or not they actually fall ill or develop clinical signs and symptoms at the time. Unwelcome though that hypothesis may be, in the chapters that follow I will present a substantial body of both clinical and experimental evidence that appears to support it, in the hope that more definitive studies will be mounted to validate or refute it.

In the case of the live-virus vaccines, it is not difficult to imagine how such a long-term carrier state might take place. It is well-known that chicken pox, herpes zoster, herpes simplex, and other live viruses are capable of surviving indefinitely for many years in a subclinical state by attaching themselves to the genetic material of their host cells, and thereby commandeering their metabolism to the limited extent of replicating along with them, but remaining latent for years and even decades and provoking acute illness only months or years later, if at all.[22]

If the live viruses of the measles, mumps, rubella, chicken pox, oral polio, and rotavirus vaccines possess a similar capability to that of the wild-type chicken pox virus, presumably the cells harboring such episomes or "proviruses" will themselves come to be recognized as foreign and thus be subject to autoimmune attack by their uninfected neighbors. Such latent carrier states could then explain how attenuated live-virus vaccines can manage to survive in the body for long enough to continue eliciting antibody responses for years without instantly or necessarily provoking the corresponding acute disease.

As for the toxoids, and the killed, denatured, recombinant, and other so-called "nonliving" vaccines, the "how" question becomes still more mysterious and problematic. What we do know for sure is that these more complicated vaccines cannot survive or function antigenically in the body for long periods of time without the presence of various chemical adsorbents, fixatives, preservatives, sterilizing agents, and a variety of so-called "adjuvants," virtually all of them highly toxic, and that enabling such long-term survival is indeed their sole purpose; but the precise mechanisms by which these carrier states are achieved are as yet poorly understood, or at least seldom talked about. If the industry knows the answer, they're not telling; and for some unaccountable reason, the CDC and the FDA seem entirely content for them to keep it a well-guarded trade secret to this day.

Nevertheless, it seems clear enough that these vaccine-adjuvant complexes must also achieve broadly similar carriage, by some means or other; and in any case, as I will presently show, there is ample evidence that autoimmune phenomena regularly do in fact result from them. At the very least, medical science needs to take this all-important question seriously, to undertake the careful, unbiased research that alone can answer it, and to inform the public accordingly; it is far too important to be allowed to remain the private property of anyone.

For the moment, however, it follows from what we do know—and again it feels almost embarrassing to have to repeat—that natural immunity results from mounting an acute, vigorous response to infection, and that whatever vaccine-mediated immunity does accomplish necessarily falls far short of that goal, because the process it sets in motion is necessarily a *chronic* one, involving in effect a reprogramming of the immune system to respond chronically to vaccines, and indeed, I fear, to other antigens as well.

It therefore strikes me as dangerously misleading, if not the exact opposite of the truth, to claim that vaccines render us immune to or somehow protect us against acute diseases if in fact they merely drive the invading organisms even deeper into the interior of our bodies and cause our vital organs to harbor them chronically if not permanently instead, such that we are rendered *incapable* or at least less capable of responding acutely, not only to them, but very probably to other antigens as well, with the result that our natural, innate cellular immune responses likewise become progressively weaker, more chronic, and show less and less capacity to heal or resolve themselves.

In short, my fear is, and indeed my experience has been, that whereas the wild-type diseases produce natural immunity through a vigorous *acute* response, artificial or vaccination-mediated immunity can only be achieved by creating the equivalent of a *chronic* infection in its place. Although this line of reasoning might seem purely conjectural at this point, analogous concerns have been expressed by other experienced observers, such as the late Harold Buttram, MD, who devoted so much of his long and distinguished career to the study of vaccines:

> Bypassing the cellular immune system, current injectable vaccines are directed toward stimulating the humoral system, thus establishing it in relative dominance over the cellular system, the reverse of the natural immunologic scheme that humans evolved with. Childhood vaccine programs may be turning childhood immune systems inside out, with the humoral system being thrown into a dominant position for which it is physiologically unsuited, while cellular immunity, lacking the challenges of the minor childhood diseases of former times, may undergo progressive atrophy from disuse. Measles, mumps, rubella, and chicken pox challenged and strengthened the immunity of both epithelial and endothelial tissues and their associated organs.[23]

In any case, as I will presently show, the practical experience of a whole generation of physicians caring for vaccine-injured children, together with an impressive body of epidemiological, clinical, and basic-science research, goes a long way toward substantiating autoimmune mechanisms as a basis for how vaccines act, for how they achieve their intended effect, and indeed for whatever else they do. In any case, as far as I know, nobody has come forward with a better or even a different explanation.

SUMMARY

The ordinary febrile illnesses of childhood, especially measles, mumps, rubella, and chicken pox, are the formative experiences for the normal maturation of the immune system, the cellular and humoral components of which act in tandem to destroy and expel foreign viral and bacterial invaders from the blood. The resulting immunity is absolute, lifelong, and twofold, i.e., both specific, preventing reinfection with the same organism, and nonspecific, priming the various cellular mechanisms to respond acutely, vigorously, and as an integrated unit to other infections in the future, thereby also helping to protect against cancer and other chronic diseases later in life.

Vaccine-mediated immunity falls far short of these goals. Bypassing the normal portal of entry, it gives the live virus, bacterium, or adjuvanted fragment thereof, free access to the blood and internal organs, where it is designed to remain on a chronic basis, and indeed more or less permanently, thus producing the equivalent of a chronic, autoimmune disease, and thereby quite possibly inhibiting the immune system from responding acutely, vigorously, and effectively to other invading organisms and foreign antigens in the future.

Chapter 2

VACCINE EFFECTIVENESS

It is mainly for their dramatic success in lowering the prevalence of various acute diseases that vaccines have been so widely acclaimed, and indeed ranked among the greatest medical and public health achievements of all time. Once again, measles is the perfect example: from an annual incidence of 400,000 to 800,000 cases annually in the United States in the early 1960s, the immediate pre-vaccine era, the figure dropped sharply in the seventies, has remained below 10,000 cases annually ever since, and has fallen below 1,000 cases in most of the years after the millennium to the point where at times it seemed on the brink of disappearing altogether.[1]

SMALL MEASLES OUTBREAKS: NO BIG DEAL

No matter how it was done or how one chooses to look at it, this must indeed be acknowledged as an achievement of historic proportions, extending beyond measles itself to the concept of vaccination in general, such that anyone would naturally wonder how and why the Disneyland measles outbreak became such a big deal. After all, comparably small outbreaks have continued to occur the whole time, and will doubtless continue even if the personal-belief exemption were eliminated, as has been shown repeatedly. In a recent Chinese study, for example, over 700 small outbreaks were documented between 2009 and 2012 in a single province boasting a vaccination rate of over 99%, and over 26,000 cases in 2013 alone.[2]

So one might well ask why the manufacturers, the CDC, and the rest of the vaccine establishment didn't just declare victory over the measles and let it go at that, in which case almost everybody would have been content, and they could still have marketed as many new vaccines as they wanted, eventually mandated all or at least most of them, and continued to vaccinate 95% of the population up to the hilt with no more than a tiny fraction of the resistance that they've stirred up now.

Given the fact that measles had already evolved from a deadly pestilence into a routine disease of childhood well before the vaccine was introduced, and had thereby been tamed and rendered about as harmless as it could ever be, not to mention conferring significant long-term health benefits on all who recovered from it, it follows that there was very little need for the vaccine in the first place, in the developed world at least, except as a publicity stunt to showcase the power and utility of the vaccination concept.

VACCINES THAT HAVE PROVEN INEFFECTIVE

In much the same vein, studying the other vaccines more carefully turns up numerous instances where vaccines have not lived up to their billing, or indeed have not worked very well at all. The most obvious example is the flu vaccine, which was aggressively promoted decades ago to protect old folks in nursing homes from this highly contagious illness that can be especially severe and at times fatal among the elderly and debilitated. Although extensive pilot studies found it to be essentially ineffective for that demographic as far back as the 1980s,[3] it has since been recycled and aggressively marketed on a yearly basis to infants, children, and adults of all ages, and finally even to pregnant women, with results that have continued to be mediocre at best.[4] This is partly because the extreme mutability of the virus virtually guarantees that a different vaccine will be needed every year, the exact specifications of which cannot be known in advance, and also because the illness we all know as "the flu" is produced by many different viruses, and is by no means restricted to the influenza group for which it is named.

POLIO, REDEFINED

Another example that most people are unaware of is polio (i.e., paralytic poliomyelitis), in which case simply introducing more precise diagnostic criteria for the disease facilitated the comforting illusion that the vaccine appeared to be much more effective than it really was. In the years before Salk's injectable polio vaccine (IPV) first appeared, the dreaded diagnosis of paralytic polio was awarded very liberally, and on purely clinical grounds, to a diverse assortment of people exhibiting paralytic symptoms for at least 24 hours, the majority of whom recovered more or less completely in a few days or weeks.

In 1954, the same year that the IPV was introduced, the CDC abruptly redefined "paralytic polio" much more narrowly, to apply to only the most severe cases in which paralysis continued for at least 60 days,[5] so that once laboratory identification of polioviruses became practical, it seemed clear, as Dr. Suzanne Humphries has recently pointed out, that in addition to milder cases of polio itself, a sizable number of the former group almost certainly included a variety of other paralytic ailments, such as Coxsackie and other enterovirus infections; poisoning with neurotoxins such as lead, arsenic, and DDT; transverse myelitis; other types of viral or "aseptic" meningitis; and Guillain-Barré syndrome.[6]

In 1969, Herbert Ratner, MD, and his colleagues compiled a report for the Illinois State Medical Society, documenting a steep decline in paralytic polio from 21,269 cases in 1952 to 7,911 in 1956; but they were very scrupulous in attributing most of it to having excluded the milder cases, rather than the action of the vaccine.[7] In any case, whether intentionally or not, the public was led to believe that the vaccine had caused these dramatic reductions, when in fact the disease had already been cut down to size by introducing these far more restrictive criteria for its diagnosis, a sleight of hand that the CDC certainly did nothing to publicize or correct, perhaps in part to avoid having to admit that the disease had always been much less prevalent than the anxious parents of that generation, including mine, understandably feared it to be.[8]

VACCINES AGAINST DISEASES ALREADY IN DECLINE

To be judged effective, vaccines need only satisfy two narrow objectives, namely,

1. a prolonged and substantial increase in the serum concentration of specific antibodies against the virus or bacterium in question, and
2. a major reduction in the incidence, morbidity, and mortality of the disease(s) it is directed against.

It turns out that these simplistic criteria are both defective, at least as much for what they leave out as for what they emphasize. The first and most obvious omission is that many of the most serious diseases that we vaccinate against were already in precipitous decline long before vaccines were developed against them. A notable example is pertussis, or whooping cough, the whole-cell vaccine against which was first introduced in 1942, a time when the falling incidence and severity of the disease led the epidemiologist C. C. Dauer to observe: "If the mortality from pertussis continues to decline at the present rate during the next fifteen years, it will be extremely difficult to show statistically that pertussis immunization had any effect in reducing the mortality from whooping cough."[9]

Much the same was true of diphtheria and tetanus, which today are almost nonexistent in the United States, except for occasional small outbreaks of the former here and there, and rare sporadic cases of the latter, mainly in the elderly; it is now generally accepted that their decline had at least as much to do with improvements in public health, hygiene, and sanitation as with vaccines and medical care.

VACCINES AGAINST MILD OR NONTHREATENING DISEASES

At the other extreme lie the diseases that are not now and never have been very serious to begin with, at least not in the developed world, such as chicken pox, which is typically so mild in young children that as late as 1996 even the American Academy of Pediatrics, that redoubtable bastion of the "vaccine establishment," advocated letting them acquire it in order to avoid the serious complications more often seen in adults.[10]

In the wake of mandatory vaccination against the disease, chicken pox has inevitably attacked growing numbers of adolescents and adults both young and old as their artificial immunity waned, precisely the state of affairs that the vaccine was introduced to prevent, as well as engineering a wholly predictable explosion of shingles and post-herpetic neuralgia among the middle-aged and elderly.

Another telling example is rotavirus, the most frequent cause of infectious diarrhea in the United States, which is responsible for many deaths among malnourished African infants and children, but rarely fatal in the developed world; vaccination is nevertheless widely used and even mandated in this country, simply because we can afford the manufacturers' hefty asking price whereas the African kids who arguably need it cannot. As the CDC freely admits, both the chicken pox and rotavirus vaccines have been mandated largely for economic reasons, and their record of accomplishment against these diseases looks a lot less impressive when measured against the nonthreatening scenarios that would almost certainly have occurred had they simply been allowed to run their course with the aid of good, old-fashioned medical care, not to mention the benefits of lifelong natural immunity that we've already discussed. In short, a case could perhaps be made for offering these vaccines and others of the same type to parents who want them; but it is a very weak one, and certainly not compelling enough to justify requiring them of everyone.

VACCINES PROMOTING MUTANT STRAINS OF THE ORIGINAL DISEASES

An even more fundamental reason for discounting the narrow official claims of vaccine efficacy is the obvious but unfashionable truth that, precisely to the extent of their success in inhibiting the spread of particular viruses and bacteria, vaccines inevitably accelerate the evolution of new mutant strains of these and related organisms, by the same law of natural selection that guarantees the proliferation of resistant forms of bacteria from the overuse of antibiotics.

This phenomenon is perhaps most readily appreciated in the case of the killed, conjugate bacterial vaccines directed against *Haemophilus influenzae* type B, or Hib, and the "pneumococcus" (i.e., *Streptococcus pneumoniae*), both of which are part of the normal flora inhabiting the nasopharynx and upper respiratory tract of most healthy people, share virtually identical capsular polysaccharide antigens, and have been associated with sporadic cases and small outbreaks of a similar array of invasive diseases in young children, including sinusitis, otitis media, epiglottitis, pneumonia, meningitis, pericarditis, and endocarditis.

First introduced in the 1970s to protect the elderly in crowded nursing homes from developing pneumonia, the pneumococcal vaccine, like the influenza vaccine, proved to be equally ineffective in a high-risk subpopulation of middle-aged and elderly veterans with significant chronic disease.[11] In the 1990s, despite this inauspicious beginning, the vaccine was recycled for pediatric use when the Finnish Otitis Media Study found it to be moderately effective in preventing ear infections, in which the pneumococcus has long played a major role.[12] But the *New England Journal of Medicine*, which published the article, promptly received a spate of letters from practicing pediatricians criticizing the study, like one pointing out that the vaccine covered only a few serotypes, and that others had already arisen to take their place.[13]

The Hib vaccine has had a similar effect, downgrading the serotypes covered by the vaccine, promoting the emergence of other serotypes, and thus altering the microecology of the normal flora in ways that will take decades to be clear about, not to mention the possibility of favoring the emergence of new, invasive diseases that have not yet appeared or been identified.

In analogous fashion, pertussis-like infections have also registered a substantial comeback in recent years, amounting to nearly 50,000 cases in the United States in 2013, the most since 1955, almost all affecting people who had previously been vaccinated.[14] The serology of these has included both pertactin-negative strains, against which the vaccine is less effective;[15] pertactin-positive or wild-type strains; and *Bordetella parapertussis*, a completely different organism that produces a similar illness but is resistant to the vaccine.[16] A powerful surface antigen, pertactin appears to be implicated significantly in the pathogenesis of wild-type whooping cough, so that the emergence of serious cases due to pertactin-negative strains clearly represents an ominous adaptation to the vaccine.

Even more disturbing is the revelation that many of these recent cases were transmitted silently from recently vaccinated carriers showing no symptoms whatsoever,[17] which has fortunately helped to discredit the long-standing official myth that unvaccinated kids are the ones to blame for the resurgence.

Although similarly downplayed, recent research has demonstrated even more clearly that the attenuated live-virus vaccines, notably MMR, varicella, rotavirus, and influenza, likewise undergo shedding in the weeks immediately following vaccination, and are thus transmissible to others and capable of spreading disease silently,[18] as is only logical, a long-overdue finding that should help discredit the widespread finger-pointing, shaming, and bullying of the unvaccinated kids and their parents as selfish and inconsiderate of their neighbors.

Over and above this transmission, the same live-virus vaccines have also engendered and helped spread completely new variants, with polio once again a major example. Although used successfully for decades throughout the world, the record of the oral polio vaccine was complicated by the shedding of live viruses, back mutations to virulence, and a significant number of paralytic cases in close contacts of the vaccinees, which led the industrialized countries to revert to the injectable version.

In the Third World, where the inexpensive OPV has remained in use, a new disease known as non-polio acute flaccid paralysis (NPAFP), which is clinically more or less identical to but even more deadly than polio, has recently emerged as a major public health threat,[19] while in the United States, which now uses IPV exclusively, a new strain of closely related enteroviruses has been isolated from a large number of patients exhibiting a disconcertingly similar picture of acute flaccid paralysis.[20] Although the vaccination status of these people has never been made public, the all-but-universal acceptance of IPV makes it a very safe bet that virtually all of them had received it, and that the new virus represents a mutant strain capable of occupying the niche vacated by its predecessor.

No less predictably, a slightly different issue has come to haunt the varicella or chicken pox vaccine, which became mandatory in 1996, in spite of many warnings that requiring it on a mass scale would weaken the immunity that would have resulted from acquiring the natural disease, and thus promote a subsequent increase in the incidence of shingles (herpes zoster) another form of the virus, which indeed has already occurred, with large numbers of shingles cases developing at progressively younger ages.[21]

Similar concerns surround the human papilloma virus (HPV) vaccines, which are currently directed only against strains 16 and 18, the two serotypes most often linked to cervical cancer, and will thus predictably succeed at least in shifting the epidemiology of that disease to other strains in the future. In addition, industry-funded studies have rather inconveniently shown that the specific antibodies resulting from natural infection with the papilloma virus are actually *protective* against cervical cancer,[22] and that the vaccine fails to prevent high-grade cervical dysplasia, widely known as the precancerous lesion that the Pap smear was designed to detect.[23]

In short, the predictable role of vaccination in manipulating and accelerating the evolutionary process in the viruses and bacteria they are targeted against represents a major obstacle to their success that has been allowed to remain more or less invisible by failing to make use of a wider, more holistic perspective on the larger microbial ecosystem that these organisms actually inhabit.

ANTIBODY TITERS DON'T MEASURE IMMUNE STATUS

As a footnote to the debate about vaccine effectiveness that should be taking place, but isn't, another important but as yet largely neglected problem is the inaccuracy of the specific antibody titer as a standard for measuring it, which has led to a multitude of tragic miscalculations. The background for this statement is the well-known fact that no vaccine is completely effective, so that all of the diseases we vaccinate against have continued to break out to some extent even in highly vaccinated populations, where the vast majority of the cases have necessarily occurred mostly among the vaccinated. As we saw, this is already visible, irrefutable, and quantitatively precise baseline evidence as to the limit of their effectiveness.

Ironically, it is also part of the reason why, instead of simply claiming victory and letting it go at that, the industry, the CDC, and their physician-allies have generally used these so-called "vaccine failures" to argue for additional "booster" shots, based on the rationale

1. that they represent essentially "bad batches" and nothing more;
2. that low titers in vaccinees mean that the vaccine immunity has "worn off," leaving behind nothing but a blank slate, such that the antibody level can be ratcheted back up to the desired level more or less at will simply by adding more shots, with the implication that the attempt to do so is entirely harmless, and that the antibody titer or concentration is an accurate measure of immune status, of the extent to which the individual is either susceptible or resistant to infection with the natural disease.

But there is ample clinical and epidemiological evidence that every one of these assumptions is false, and that as a result, our understanding of how vaccines really act inside the human body and how they accomplish whatever it is that they accomplish is fundamentally mistaken, and requires a completely different perspective that looks at the procedure much more broadly and deeply than our present set of blinders seem to allow.

In the first place, it has been known for quite a long time that the antibody titer cannot be manipulated at will by simply adding more boosters to the schedule. As far back as 1980, James Cherry, MD, then as now a leading vaccine advocate, showed quite conclusively that children previously vaccinated against the measles whose specific antibody titers had fallen below supposedly immune levels responded only minimally and for an unacceptably short time to a booster shot.[24]

Both the outbreaks of measles in fully vaccinated populations and the failure of Cherry's booster shot to remain effective for an extended period already cast doubt on the conventional wisdom that immunity is a purely quantitative variable, that the specific antibody titer accurately measures it, and that by applying sufficient chemical force it can be increased to the desired level more or less at will. Nevertheless, major outbreaks of the measles over the ensuing years generated intense pressure to do something about them, such that Cherry's research was discreetly shelved, the MMR booster was duly mandated for all children, and it remains in force to this day.[25]

An even more suggestive finding emerged from a sustained outbreak of 235 cases in Wisconsin, over a nine-month period in 1986.[26] In addition to the usual cases, of whom 94% were vaccinated, the authors identified a large subset of what they called "mild measles," consisting of a much paler rash, no fever, and minimal discomfort, fatigue, or other systemic involvement.[27] To their considerable surprise, they discovered that this syndrome was much more common in vaccinated kids with no antibodies whatsoever, while the florid, acute illness was seen not only in the unvaccinated kids, as expected, but also in vaccinated kids with high and supposedly immune levels of antibodies.[28]

This paradoxical finding indicated some kind of latent viral activity in vaccinated patients that had gone undetected, and was in fact belied by routine serological testing. It raised the disturbing possibility that vaccinees showing very low or zero titers were being mistakenly identified as susceptible, inappropriately revaccinated, and thus put at risk of developing more serious reactions as a result.

A few years later, I happened to witness just such a misfortune when called upon to file a VICP report on behalf of a young patient who had submitted a claim for damages after suffering a prolonged respiratory ailment from her first round of Hep B vaccines, followed by chronic, autoimmune thyroiditis after the second:

> A previously healthy 31-year-old lab technician developed autoimmune thyroiditis soon after her second round of Hep B vaccinations. At 24 her doctor gave her the first round, as required for her training, beginning with two shots two months apart; soon after the second dose, she developed a severe, persistent cough that lasted for weeks and finally cleared up on antibiotics, after which she took the third shot, with no apparent reaction.
>
> But four years later, when her new employer retested her, he found no specific antibodies at all, concluded that she was still susceptible, and insisted that she receive a second round. Within a few days after the first dose, she developed a sore throat and cold symptoms, followed by weakness, fatigue, hoarseness, and weight gain, all of which persisted for months.
>
> Although she managed to delay the second dose for quite a long time, she nevertheless worsened immediately after it, with an even more intense version of the same cough she had had in the past, this time accompanied by palpitations and anxiety at night. Finding her TSH elevated to twice the normal level, her doctor gave her thyroid hormone, followed by a third dose of Hep B, after which both her symptoms and her elevated TSH persisted for months with no improvement. At this point anti-thyroid antibodies were found, and she continued to worsen, despite ever-higher doses of hormone and normal thyroid-

function tests. She has since developed a nodular goiter, difficulty swallowing, and esophageal reflux.

In short, this previously healthy young woman remains chronically ill as a result of her Hep B vaccinations, and will almost certainly need regular medical supervision and treatment for the rest of her life.[29]

The most clear-cut of any of the several Hep B vaccine cases that I've reviewed for the VICP, her claim was dismissed without a hearing according to current federal guidelines, which fail to acknowledge any causal link between vaccines and ongoing autoimmune or indeed chronic diseases of any type, much less any silent viral activity in vaccinees of the kind that her case seems to point to.

SUMMARY

The flu vaccine stands for a sizable number of others that have not been effective, even by their own standards. In addition, the criteria for vaccine effectiveness need to be reevaluated. First, the observed decline in incidence of the corresponding natural diseases is often misleading,

1. because many were already in decline (e.g., pertussis);
2. because some were redefined much more narrowly (e.g., polio);
3. because viral and bacterial shedding cause outbreaks among vaccinees (live viruses, pertussis, Hib, and pneumococcus); and
4. because new strains and serotypes emerge by natural selection (polio, pertussis, Hib, pneumococcus, chicken pox, HPV).

Second, specific antibody titers don't measure immune status accurately, resulting in both false positives (outbreaks in highly vaccinated populations) and false negatives (boosters ineffective, and patients with zero titers developing even worse disease when revaccinated), indicating unsuspected latent viral activity.

Chapter 3

VACCINE SAFETY

The issue of vaccine safety is unavoidably controversial and indeed highly polarized, pitting repeated assurances from manufacturers, government agencies, and physicians that vaccines are uniformly safe against thousands upon thousands of injured children put forward as living proof by their parents that they are not. On the face of it, they cannot both be right. Safety is thus inescapably a core issue that needs to be settled, one way or the other.

VACCINES ARE DRUGS

Whatever else it may claim to be, the ingestion or inoculation of live bacteria, viruses, or their killed, denatured, or genetically engineered derivatives for the purpose of preventing or minimizing the risk of the corresponding infections is ultimately a form of medical treatment like any other, involving the administration of powerful pharmaceutical drugs with the advertised capacity to achieve a certain physiological result.

From that fact alone, it follows as the night the day that, in some proportion to their chemical power and causal effectiveness, they necessarily pose certain health risks for the recipient. This much, I think, both sides can agree on; and if so, the question ultimately boils down to one of *numbers*, rather than simply yes or no, and includes not only what adverse reactions can occur, and how serious they are, but also *how often* they occur.

Secondly, the industry and the CDC might even agree that the public has the right to be informed about these risks, utilizing the most sophisticated tools and methods of scientific investigation available, and to weigh them carefully against the benefits anticipated from their use, just as with all other drugs.

Naturally, the industry has already conducted its own safety trials for each vaccine; and both their design and rules of conduct are conveniently summarized in the package inserts accompanying each one, which have been collected in the *Physicians' Desk Reference*, or *PDR*, and thus provide the obvious starting point for any such inquiry.

Of course, vaccines are also commercial products; so the package inserts contain only the data that the manufacturers see fit to disclose, and are couched in the technical jargon of the industry. Some reading between the lines is therefore necessary, both to translate what they say into plain language and to notice what they leave unsaid. But carefully encrypted within them lies a surprisingly rich storehouse of valuable information.

NO UNTREATED PLACEBO CONTROLS

To begin with, even without a scientific background, anyone already curious about these safety trials is apt to be disturbed by the virtually complete *absence* of something we have all come to expect, namely, a control group of untreated individuals for comparison. This omission is both glaring and problematic, first, because by current standards it becomes impossible to establish a genuine cause-and-effect relationship between the vaccine and whatever adverse reactions are observed after giving it, and second, because that result was intentional.

In 2012, in response to persistent interrogation before a Congressional Committee, Dr. Colleen Boyle, a senior CDC official, reluctantly admitted under oath that the CDC, the FDA, the NIH, and the manufacturers themselves routinely avoid using unvaccinated controls as a matter of policy,[1] a radical departure from this widely accepted "gold standard" of biomedical research.

With ActHIB, Sanofi-Pasteur's Hib vaccine, for example, the subjects receiving the Hib were given the DTP vaccine also, while the so-called "controls" received both the DTP and either the oral polio or the hepatitis B for comparison.[2] In other words, the study addresses the comparative risk of different groups of vaccines, but says nothing about the risk of death or serious adverse reactions from the Hib vaccine alone, which is what parents, physicians, and scientists would naturally want to know.[3] The only answer we get is the reassurance that deaths and serious or life-threatening complications were not significantly more frequent after the Hib and DTP vaccines than for the other combinations.

As for these complications, which included urticaria, seizures, renal failure, and Guillain-Barré syndrome, or GBS, a crippling and sometimes fatal polyneuropathy, we are told only that "a cause-and-effect relationship with the vaccine has not been established,"[4] and left to figure out for ourselves that, without a placebo-control group for comparison, a causal relationship could *never* be established, no matter how many deaths or adverse reactions occurred.

Simply asking why this was done then prompts a second question, namely, why the DTP was added to both groups in the first place. A much older product featuring the whole-cell pertussis vaccine, the DTP was taken off the market decades ago because of the large number of court settlements for brain damage that had resulted from its mandated use in the 1980s and 1990s. Sanofi-Pasteur's curious resurrection of it here immediately arouses suspicion that its dismal safety record might have been made use of to conceal the adverse reactions to both the Hib and hepatitis B vaccines inside the even larger total of bad outcomes to be expected from the DTP.

As it happens, the same manufacturer also used the DTP in another such "control" group to evaluate the safety of the DTaP vaccine that they developed to replace it, featuring the presumably safer acellular pertussis component.[5] Once again, the study merely shows that the new product was safer than the old, not that it was safe in any absolute sense,[6] and thus amounts to little more than advertising to promote its sale by touting it above its rivals, aided by the further incentive that the study was conducted by the prestigious National Institutes of Health, the premier investigative agency of the federal government.

With very few exceptions, almost all vaccine safety studies are likewise conducted without a control group of unvaccinated individuals receiving nothing but an inert placebo. In the case of Gardasil, Merck's highly touted HPV vaccine, the manufacturer employed an even more devious strategy that has also proved widely popular in the industry.

To provoke a long-lasting antibody response in their recipients, Gardasil and many other vaccines contain aluminum salts as an adjuvant; so for comparison with the experimental group receiving Gardasil, the Merck scientists devised two so-called "control" groups, namely, (1) a small one (n=320 subjects) receiving genuine placebo (i.e., saline alone), and (2) a much larger one (n=3,470 subjects), roughly comparable to the Gardasil group, receiving only the aluminum adjuvant,[7] even though the adjuvant is a known neurotoxin, which has been causally linked to several varieties of brain damage, and has thus become a main focus of independent research into the health risks of the many vaccines that contain it.

For minor adverse effects, as expected, the small group receiving inert placebo suffered proportionally far fewer adverse effects than either of the other two; but for more serious and life-threatening reactions, it was arbitrarily mixed into the larger population receiving the aluminum adjuvant. This combined group was then compared with the group of similar size receiving Gardasil, without revealing the different rates of complications between those receiving the adjuvant and those receiving saline alone.[8]

Because the much lower number and rate of deaths and serious and life-threatening complications to be expected in the tiny saline-placebo group were insignificant compared to those in the vastly larger group receiving the aluminum, they became essentially invisible, so that the risk of serious adverse events for the combined groups came out roughly the same as that for the group receiving Gardasil. Precisely that result was documented in the subset of girls and women of ages 9 through 26, with each group showing a comparable and indeed substantial incidence of well over a hundred cases of various autoimmune diseases, many of them serious,[9] while in default of any other explanation we must assume that the concealment was intentional.

INADEQUATE SUPERVISION

Another important but often neglected aspect of how clinical trials are designed and conducted is the manner in which the subjects are supervised, which can play a decisive role in framing, shaping, and thus influencing their outcome. Once again, the Gardasil insert provides a tantalizingly incomplete but still revealing answer. Subjects received Gardasil, aluminum adjuvant, or saline, respectively, on the day of enrollment, and again 2 months and 6 months thereafter, for a total of 3 injections, and were told to keep report cards for 14 days after each one, at which point they were interviewed about them.[10]

Limiting the observation period to three widely separated periods of 14 days each already casts serious doubt on the results, because a primary antibody response to an antigen encountered for the first time requires at least 14 days; and in my experience it can easily take longer than that, weeks or even months, for serious chronic conditions to develop and manifest. The obvious and inevitable result, if not the intent, of limiting the study period to 14 days after each dose is thus to exclude almost all chronic diseases from consideration purely arbitrarily, as a matter of policy.

Based on that guideline, complications appearing at times when the subjects were not being observed, even if still occurring in the next observation period, could then be easily interpreted and written off as coincidental (i.e., due to a preexisting condition or tendency), and thus unrelated to the vaccine. To make a true assessment of the safety risks of any vaccine, then, what we need to know is

1. how many deaths and serious adverse effects were recorded in each of the groups listed separately;
2. how many deaths and serious complications were actually reported by the subjects themselves or their families;
3. what criteria the investigator in charge of the study used to decide which ones were attributable to the vaccine and which were not; and
4. how many of the reported complications were listed as "vaccine-related," and how many were thrown out (i.e., attributed to "coincidence" or some other cause).

As it happens, the package inserts have a good deal to say regarding point 4, but provide contradictory data for 2, and are completely silent as to 1 and 3. With Gardasil, we learn that only 0.04% of the serious adverse reactions reported by the subjects themselves were judged to be vaccine-related by the lead investigator.[11]

In short, we are asked to believe that 99.96% of all the serious adverse reactions reported by the subjects themselves throughout the study period had nothing to do with the vaccine and could therefore be dismissed from the tally. One can only marvel at how Merck had the audacity to publish such a statistic, let alone how they've managed to avoid independent scrutiny of it for so long, or why, if not purely for appearances' sake, the subjects were asked to keep detailed "vaccination report cards," if only 4 in 10,000 of their most serious complaints were deemed credible or worthy of inclusion in the study. Truly, it boggles the mind.

THE LEAD INVESTIGATOR GETS TO DECIDE

As to the basis for these determinations, we are told only that the subjects handed in their report cards at the end of each 14-day observation period, at which point the lead investigator made a determination, yes or no, based on criteria about which we are told nothing whatsoever.

To be sure, in a well-run society, we would have every reason to trust the scientists who work on our behalf to execute such judgments fairly, without bias or any prior agenda determining the outcome; but the manufacturers' penchant for keeping mum about their actual procedures lends still further credence to the suspicion that the lead investigator's main assignment is to do whatever is necessary to ensure that the results of such trials conform to the company's predetermined agenda of advertising the product to be as safe and effective as possible.

As it happens, an insider with expert, firsthand knowledge of the industry recently made no bones of the fact that this worst-case scenario is actually Standard Operating Procedure throughout the industry. In a documentary about the HPV vaccine, Dr. Peter Rost, a former vice president of Pfizer, catalogued in minute detail the aggressive marketing strategies that he himself devised and oversaw to promote his company's products, which, although in flagrant violation of the ethical guidelines Pfizer still publicly subscribes to, were nevertheless the usual practice throughout the industry, as indeed they still remain:

> Universities, health organizations, and everybody is out there begging for money. Nobody has any money. The only ones who do are the big international corporations, and they have lots of money. They give grants for research, pay doctors and researchers thousands of dollars to travel around, speak at conferences, and establish educational programs, all in order to make profits for their products. [The safety trials] are supposedly third-party and independent, but the money won't keep coming unless they support your drug, unless they say what you want them to say. Everybody knows that this is how things work. The drug companies know it, and you know it; only the public doesn't know it.[12]

As for the other vaccines, a careful perusal of their safety studies lays bare a repertoire of methodologies that take precisely similar liberties with accepted standards of valid biomedical research, utilizing much the same repertoire of deceptions and ambiguities that we have just described. In particular,

1. the vast majority of studies involve defective control groups receiving either a different vaccine or vaccines, or the highly reactive adjuvant alone, while the few that claim to employ placebo controls are limited to much smaller groups, and the actual content of these "placebos" is not specified;
2. the observation period is very brief and tightly restricted, with the result that only a tiny, insignificant fraction of the deaths and serious adverse events reported by the subjects are actually attributed to the vaccine; and

3. the lead investigator is given extraordinary latitude to decide whether or not the serious adverse reactions reported are vaccine-related, based on criteria that are never specified.

Adverse Reactions, Solicited and Unsolicited

With many of the newer vaccines, an additional distinction is made between

4. the small number of "solicited" adverse reactions previously named by the investigator and specifically asked about during the brief monitoring period, rarely exceeding 14 days after each shot, and typically separated by intervals of at least several months between them; and
5. the large wastebasket category of unsolicited reports of serious adverse reactions reported by the subjects themselves or their parents over a longer period, which have to be submitted according to strict rules, and are subject to review by the investigator, who then decides that they are or are not vaccine-related, according to criteria about which once again we are told nothing at all.

The following is an alphabetical list of the other currently mandated vaccines, with a brief summary of controlled studies, if any, and monitoring procedures:

1. **DTaP vaccine** (Adacel, Sanofi-Pasteur):
   No controlled studies;
   Adverse reactions asked about for 14 days after each shot;
   ER, hospital visits, and serious illnesses tracked for 6 months;
   Unsolicited phone reports accepted for review for 6 months.[13]

2. **Flu vaccine, Quadrivalent** (Fluarix, GlaxoSmithKline):
   Controls get mono-, di-, or trivalent versions of the Sanofi-Pasteur vaccine;
   Solicited adverse reactions asked about for 7 days after each shot;
   Unsolicited reports accepted for review if submitted within 21 days.[14]

3. **Hepatitis B vaccine** (Engerix, GlaxoSmithKline):
   No controlled studies;
   Solicited adverse reactions asked about for 4 days after each shot;
   No information about unsolicited reports.[15]

4. **Hepatitis B vaccine** (Recombivax HB, Merck):
   No controlled studies; one group gets 2 doses, the other gets 3;
   Solicited adverse reactions asked about for 5 days after each shot;
   No information about unsolicited reports.[16]

5. **Hib Conjugate vaccine** (Hiberix, GlaxoSmithKline):
   Subjects get Hiberix plus DTaP and Hep B, IPV, or both;
   Controls get Merck, Wyeth, or Sanofi-Pasteur Hib vaccine, plus DTaP and Hep B, IPV, or both;
   Solicited adverse reactions asked about for 4 days after each shot;
   No information about unsolicited reports.[17]

6. **Hib Liquid Conjugate vaccine** (Pedvax, Merck):
   Subjects also get DTP and OPV;
   Controls get lyophilized version plus DTP and OPV;
   Solicited adverse reactions asked about for 3 days after each shot;
   No information about unsolicited reports.[18]

7. **HPV vaccine** (Cervarix, GlaxoSmithKline):
   Control groups get single or double dose of hepatitis A vaccine;
   Solicited adverse reactions asked about for 7 days after each shot;
   Unsolicited reports accepted for review if submitted within 30 days.[19]

8. **Measles, Mumps, and Rubella vaccine** (MMR II (Merck):
   No safety studies, just postmarketing surveillance (VAERS reports).[20]

9. **Pneumococcal vaccine, 23-valent** (Pneumovax 23,Merck):
   Controls get "placebo," i.e., phenol 0.25%.
   Solicited adverse reactions asked about for 5 days after each shot.
   No information about unsolicited reports.[21]

10. **Pneumococcal vaccine, 7-valent** (Prevnar, Wyeth-Pfizer):
    No randomized, controlled studies: various groups get other vaccines;
    Solicited adverse reactions asked about by phone at 48 hours;
    ER and hospital visits tracked at 3, 14, and 30 days;
    Long-term follow-up at 1 year by VAERS reports.[22]

11. **Pneumococcal vaccine, 13-valent** (Prevnar-13, Wyeth-Pfizer):
    Controls get Prevnar 7-valent): 4 shots given, 2, 4, 6, 12–15 months;
    Solicited adverse reactions asked about for 7 days after each shot;
    Unsolicited reports accepted for review if submitted at any time during the study period, or by phone interview after fourth dose, and again 6 months after that.[23]

12. **Polio vaccine, inactivated** (IPV: IPOL, Sanofi-Pasteur):
    Subjects get IPOL and DTP at 2, 4, and 18 months; controls get DTP alone;
    Solicited adverse reactions asked about for 48 hours after each shot;
    No information about unsolicited reports.[24]

13. **Rotavirus vaccine** (Rotarix, GlaxoSmithKline):
    Controls get unspecified "placebo";
    Solicited adverse reactions asked about for 7 days after each dose;
    No information about unsolicited reports.[25]

14. **Rotavirus vaccine** (RotaTeq, Merck):
    Controls get unspecified "placebo";
    Solicited reactions asked about at 7, 14, and 42 days after each dose;
    Unsolicited reports accepted for review if submitted within 42 days.[26]

15. **Varicella vaccine** (Varivax, Merck):
    Controls get unspecified "placebo";
    Subjects and controls "actively followed" for 42 days.[27]

16. **Zoster or shingles vaccine** (Zostavax, Merck):
    Controls get unspecified "placebo";
    Solicited adverse reactions asked about for 5 days after each shot;
    Unsolicited reports accepted for review if submitted from report cards within 42 days, or by monthly phone interviews for 2–5 years thereafter.[28]

The important detail to keep in mind is that the "solicited" adverse reactions identified in advance and specifically asked about by the investigator represent the very few that have been accepted and made official by the industry and the CDC, like anaphylaxis, or intussusception in the case of rotavirus. The fact that such a distinction was made by some manufacturers but not others, and quite recently at that, suggests that they agreed to review the unsolicited reports of adverse reactions submitted by the subjects themselves only reluctantly, in response to protests from the latter that their complaints were not being taken seriously.

In any case, the distinction provides no real benefit to the subjects. What it does accomplish is simply to institutionalize and legitimize the industry's customary practice of accepting the very small number of solicited reactions more or less automatically as "caused" by the vaccine, and indeed as the bulk of adverse reactions admitted into the study, while the much larger number of unsolicited reports by the subjects and their parents, many of which fall outside the period of close monitoring, are easily relegated to a broad wastebasket category that the investigator is entirely free and indeed highly likely to reject as idiosyncratic hypersensitivity reactions based on a preexisting latent tendency, and therefore coincidental or unrelated to the vaccine.

Another reason for suspecting that this unstated triage guideline is partly responsible for the implausibly low rate of serious adverse reactions tallied in these studies is how closely it matches the clinical criteria that both practicing physicians and the VAERS and VICP systems habitually use in evaluating the claims of injured vaccinees and their parents in the real world, which are minimized by widespread underreporting, to begin with, and are rarely successful in any case, as we shall see.

THE HELSINKI DECLARATION AND THE NUREMBERG CODE

The absence of unvaccinated controls in vaccine safety studies merits special attention, because it poses a further threat to the basic human right of informed consent that the policy of mandatory vaccination seeks to override. This right was promulgated in what is known as the Helsinki Declaration, "Ethical Principles for Medical Research Involving Human Subjects," an extension of the 1947 Nuremberg Code, both of which were incorporated into international law in the wake of Nazi atrocities in World War II.

Explaining in her Congressional testimony that it would be unethical to leave any children unprotected against vaccine-preventable diseases, Dr. Colleen Boyle of the CDC invoked a provision in the original Declaration that allows for the use of placebo controls only if there is no treatment proven effective for the condition, and if the use of placebo, by withholding such treatment, would not impose a substantial risk of irreversible harm:

> The use of placebo, or no treatment, is acceptable in studies where no proven intervention exists, or where for compelling and scientifically sound methodological reasons the use of placebo is necessary to determine the efficacy or safety of an intervention, and the patients who receive placebo or no treatment will not be subject to any risk of serious or irreversible harm.[29]

Evidently, Dr. Boyle is relying on the Declaration's scrupulous wording, which appears to restrict the use of placebo-controlled trials to certain special circumstances (i.e., as an exception rather than the rule). But her argument breaks down on closer reading of the document as a whole, which makes it clear that its hesitation regarding the use of placebo controls would rarely if ever apply to vaccine research, for several reasons.

First, the studies that allegedly prove vaccinations to be a safe and effective treatment are themselves profoundly flawed, as we have seen, while placebo-controlled trials have long since become the "gold standard" for establishing a causal relationship between *any* drug or medical procedure and the signs and symptoms that follow its use, whether intended or not, and are therefore the best technique that is currently available for determining vaccine safety and efficacy.

Second, vaccines are not given to *treat* anything, but merely to prevent a possible illness in the indefinite future, which the subject might never actually encounter, and which might not be serious even then, whereas the spirit of the Declaration rules out the use of placebo controls solely in the exceptional circumstance of serious or potentially fatal diseases, either already present or imminently threatening, that would pose a substantial threat to life and limb if left untreated.

And third, many of the thousands of parents who chose not to vaccinate would gladly volunteer their children to serve as the control group for such studies, in which case nobody would have to be deprived of anything or forced to submit to anything against their will, since they have already made and unequivocally declared their choice.

The overriding importance of free choice and the informed consent of the participants is likewise emphasized in the very first article of the Nuremberg Code of 1947, in reaction to the inhuman medical experiments conducted in Nazi death and concentration camps, and upon which the Helsinki Declaration itself was explicitly based: "Required is the voluntary, well-informed, understanding consent of the human subject in a full legal capacity."[30]

Free choice and informed consent are of central importance in the Helsinki Declaration as well, since whether to waive or allow placebo controls would ultimately turn on the subject's or parent's own preference as to need and risk, which in a doubtful or ambiguous case would clearly trump any narrowly technical and methodological issues:

> In medical research involving competent human subjects, each potential subject must be adequately informed of the aims, methods, sources of funding, any possible conflicts of interest, institutional affiliations of the researcher, anticipated benefits and potential risks of the study and the discomfort it may entail, and any other relevant aspects of the study.
>
> The potential subject must be informed of the right to refuse to participate in the study or to withdraw consent to participate at any time without reprisal. After ensuring that the potential subject has understood the information, the physician or another appropriately qualified individual must then seek the potential subject's freely given informed consent, preferably in writing.[31]

THE INADEQUACIES OF INDUSTRY-FUNDED DRUG RESEARCH

Thanks to the inaccurate and false assumptions built into these trials, we really do not know the full extent of deaths and serious adverse reactions to vaccines; and if the present system is allowed to continue, it is clear that we never will. But what is beyond doubt is that the true figures are considerably higher, perhaps as much as several orders of magnitude higher, than those provided by the industry.

In addition, the pervasiveness of these unethical carryings-on has engendered a growing distrust of the entire medical research enterprise, to a degree that would have been unthinkable a generation ago, and involving some of the most highly respected voices in the profession. One such is Marcia Angell, MD, currently a professor at Harvard Medical School, whose long and illustrious career as editor of the *New England Journal of Medicine* was abruptly terminated for the unpardonable offense of bearing witness to many of the same abuses that we have just been discussing, and who has written a book and many articles highly critical of the pharmaceutical industry as a whole:

> Conflicts of interest and biases exist in virtually every field of medicine, particularly those that rely heavily on drugs or devices. It is no longer possible to believe much of the clinical research that is published, or to rely on the judgment of trusted physicians or authoritative medical guidelines. I take no pleasure in this conclusion, which I reached slowly and reluctantly over my two decades as editor of *The New England Journal of Medicine*.[32]

> The boundaries between academic medicine and the pharmaceutical industry have been dissolving since the 1980s, and the major differences between their missions are becoming blurred. Medical research, education, and clinical practice have suffered as a result.
>
> Most clinical trials are funded by the pharmaceutical industry. Since drug companies don't have direct access to human subjects, they contract with academic researchers to conduct trials on patients in teaching hospitals and clinics. Until the mid-1980s, drug companies gave grants to medical centers for researchers to test their products, waited for the results, and hoped their products looked good. Sponsors had no part in designing or analyzing the studies, and didn't claim to own the data or write papers or control publication.
>
> That distance is a thing of the past. The major drug companies are now hugely profitable; they make more in profit and spend twice as much on marketing and administration as on R & D. In contrast, medical centers have fallen on difficult times. Academic medical centers have become supplicants to the drug companies, deferring to them in ways that would have been unthinkable twenty years ago. Often academic researchers are little more than hired hands who supply human subjects and collect data according to instructions from corporate paymasters. The sponsors keep the data, analyze it, write the papers, and decide whether, when, and where to submit them for publication In multi-center trials, researchers may not even be allowed to

> see the data, an obvious impediment to science and a perversion of standard practice.
>
> Manufacturers prefer to work with academic medical centers, to increase the chances of getting research published, and provide them access to influential faculty physicians, who write textbooks and medical-journal articles, sit on government advisory panels, and speak at meetings that teach clinicians about prescription drugs.
>
> Academic researchers also have other financial ties to the companies that sponsor their work. They serve as consultants to the companies whose products they evaluate, join corporate advisory boards and speaker bureaus, enter into royalty arrangements, agree to be listed authors of articles ghostwritten by interested companies, promote drugs and devices at company-sponsored symposia, and allow themselves to be plied with expensive gifts and trips to luxurious settings. Many also have equity interest in the sponsoring companies.[33]

In short, as Dr. Angell's books and articles make clear, the issue is not between those who believe in science and those who do not, as many vaccine advocates would have us believe, but rather the inadequacy of what is allowed to pass for science these days, and the involuntary experiments, runaway profits, and invisible casualties that are so righteously justified in its name.

SUMMARY

Vaccine safety trials are almost entirely funded, conducted, and micromanaged by the manufacturers themselves, employing methods that deviate sharply from accepted scientific standards:

1. Instead of unvaccinated controls receiving inert placebo, they use control groups receiving other vaccines, or adjuvants alone;
2. They do not monitor the subjects for more than 14 days after each shot, thus excluding from consideration any adverse reactions that occur at other times (i.e., chronic illnesses);
3. They look for and take seriously the reactions that the investigator has identified in advance and specifically asks about, and are less receptive to other unsolicited reactions that the subjects report; and

4. The lead investigator then decides whether or not the reactions are vaccine-related, according to criteria that are unspecified, but typically accepting the few solicited reactions and rejecting most of the others.

These methods indicate widespread corruption at the heart of the drug industry, which is largely rubber-stamped by the regulatory agencies, in order to inflate the safety record and minimize the risks of vaccines, with the result that these studies can no longer be relied upon to provide fair, objective, unbiased evidence, and that vaccines must necessarily be reckoned as considerably more dangerous than officially acknowledged.

PART II

EVIDENCE OF HARM

Chapter 4

THE CLINICAL PERSPECTIVE

Private encounters between physicians and patients are the familiar and comfortable setting where practicing physicians like me do most of our work; and the personal relationships that develop from them are the source of our power to unlock secrets that prove impenetrable otherwise. Although its purview necessarily includes the scientific realm of abstract causes, mechanisms, diseases, and the technical language of abnormalities, the clinical perspective ultimately succeeds or fails in the concrete realm of the here-and-now, the unique, lived experience of individual human beings.

TRUSTING OUR PATIENTS

When parents tell me that their kids have been injured or made sick by vaccines or anything else, it's obviously a crucial part of my job to determine as best I can whether and to what extent that attribution is accurate; and, certainly, there have been my fair share of times when I've had good reason to believe that it isn't. But as the foundation of everything that I undertake on their behalf, my relationships with patients are necessarily built on mutual trust and respect.

By that, I don't mean that I always believe or agree with what they say, but rather that I trust what my patients tell me to be *the truth as they live it*, whether rightly or wrongly, until something happens to convince me otherwise. Indeed, experience has taught me that doctors who question and doubt the official assurances that vaccines are uniformly safe and effective have come to this position out of their commitment to honor that same assumption, while those who would mandate vaccines for everyone without exception often act as if what passes for science these days entitles them to dismiss and override the beliefs and values of patients whom they happen to dislike or disagree with.

Similar sentiments prompted the late Dr. Robert Mendelsohn, a beloved professor of pediatrics from an older generation, to insist that parents were the true experts on the health of their children, and that pediatricians who understood that were being marginalized by the extravagant claims of modern science, technology, and the giant industries that control them, in words that ring even truer today:

> Parents are better than doctors at managing their children's health. Unless you've passed the half-century mark, you can't be expected to remember the old "family doctor," for today there are very few left. Those who still can are apt to remember them with affection, as friendly, unpretentious, reassuring, and compassionate, someone intimately involved with our families for generations. He knew each of us as individuals, was sensitive to our attitudes, moods, and idiosyncrasies, and viewed us as human beings in need of help, not clinical subjects for technical and pharmacological interventions. He listened patiently, answered thoughtfully, calmed our fears, and explained simply and clearly. If we needed a pill, we got one, but more often he allayed our fears with calm reassurance and let Nature do its work without interference.
>
> I may have romanticized him, but what he was is what today's doctors should be. Unfortunately, few of them are; so it falls to you, the parents, to assume that role. How can you do it better than pediatricians? Because you're willing to give your children the time and attention, and your doctor isn't. The typical pediatrician's assembly line spews out 30 or more patients a day, doesn't know your child as you do, and has neither the time nor the inclination to learn. In most instances, all his tests, shots, and X-rays are no substitute for the common-sense care that an informed parent can provide.[1]

Founded on decades of clinical experience, this distinctly old-fashioned attitude led Dr. Mendelsohn to oppose mandatory vaccination at a time when even to question it was already considered proof of heresy:

> There is no convincing scientific evidence that mass inoculation can be credited with eliminating any childhood disease. It's true that some diseases have diminished or disappeared in the US since inoculations were introduced, but one must ask why they did so simultaneously in Europe, where mass immunization did not take place.
>
> There are significant risks associated with every immunization. Yet doctors administer them routinely without warning parents or determining whether they're contraindicated for that particular child. No one knows the long-term

> consequence of injecting foreign proteins into the body of your child, and no one is making any structured effort to find out.
>
> There is growing suspicion that immunization against relatively harmless childhood diseases may be responsible for the dramatic increase in autoimmune diseases, cancer, leukemia, rheumatoid arthritis, Lou Gehrig's Disease, lupus, and Guillain-Barré syndrome. Have we traded mumps and measles for cancer and leukemia?[2]

DOCTORS FOR SAFER VACCINES, INFORMED CONSENT, AND FULL DISCLOSURE

In the decades since Dr. Mendelsohn's book, many other clinicians have come forward voicing similar questions, doubts, and concerns—increasingly backed up by the latest scientific research, but still based on the old-fashioned heresy of trusting our patients and the clinical perspective that is based on it. What is remarkable is not only that there are so many of us out there, but also that our arguments and objections all sound so much alike, because they arise not from theory or speculation, but rather from our shared, cumulative, and hard-won experience in the trenches of everyday medical practice.

I'm thinking of people like Sherri Tenpenny, DO, a dedicated family physician who believed in vaccines and dutifully vaccinated according to the official schedule for many years, until growing doubts and fears brought her to a conference sponsored by the National Vaccine Information Center in 2000, which opened her eyes to the hidden backstory. Ever since then, she has devoted a major portion of her career to researching vaccines and writing and educating the public about them:

> I decided to go to the CDC, and discovered that most of what I'd accepted as the truth about vaccines really wasn't true at all: that vaccines weren't responsible for the eradication of polio and smallpox, and haven't been proven safe; that vaccines deemed "effective" may still not protect against the disease; that research studies use a second vaccine as placebo, not an inert substance; and that vaccines are not harmless, that many thousands have been injured and many hundreds have died as a result of them.[3]

Suzanne Humphries, MD, another physician-activist, is a board-certified nephrologist with many years of clinical experience who took care of several patients with renal failure during the 2009 flu season, and became shocked and disillusioned by the painfully obvious link between the condition and the flu vaccine, which her colleagues flatly refused to acknowledge, a dilemma that led her to give up her successful practice in favor of full-time research into how vaccines act. She has since become a leading advocate for a saner policy regarding their use:

> The most memorable event was in the winter of 2009, when the H1N1 flu vaccine was given. Three patients in close succession were wheeled into the ER with total kidney shutdown. When I talked to them, each one volunteered, "I was fine until I had that vaccine." All three had shown normal kidney function in their outpatient records, and all three required dialysis. Two recovered, and one died of complications several months later.
>
> I began taking vaccine histories on all my patients, and was often startled by what I heard. Several had been admitted with normal kidneys but had their health decline within 24 hours of the vaccine, and even these well-defined and documented cases were denied as vaccine-induced by my colleagues, except for the rare doctor or nurse who would agree with me in private, when nobody was listening. I resolved to find out everything I could about safety trials for vaccines. What I learned led me to leave my practice and become a full-time researcher on vaccination and the immune system.[4]

While in charge of the emergency department at Michael Reese Hospital in Chicago, the pediatrician Toni Bark, MD, noticed that a sizable number of kids who had recently been seen at the Vaccine Clinic were showing up at her ER with a variety of ailments, such that she, too, stopped vaccinating without parental consent, and has since become a committed and persuasive advocate for upholding the personal-belief exemption:

> Children seen in the vaccine clinic would come to our ER with seizures, respiratory arrest and asthma attacks. I began to realize that not all children respond well to vaccines, and that some die. Later I began to see the fraud and corruption in the Advisory Committees and in how vaccines are marketed.
>
> I had no idea that those killed and injured had no recourse against either manufacturer or physician. Manufacturers enjoy full immunity from lawsuits, and the Vaccine Court is almost a secret, yet has paid out $3 billion since 1986. The VAERS system is also poorly advertised, and the government admits it receives only 10% of the adverse events that occur.

> We mandate more vaccines than any other country, and have a higher infant mortality rate than some third world countries. Most kids do OK, but some don't. Genetics and timing are also important; no drug or dosage is right for everyone. Federal cases against drug companies show that safety data are hidden, manipulated, and even fabricated. Most safety studies use fake placebos, like aluminum adjuvant for HPV, or a Meningitis Vaccine for Pneumo. All independent meta-analyses say that real safety studies are needed. There are 200+ new vaccines in the pipeline, and all of them will be approved, recommended, and mandated. Isn't enough enough?
>
> After Nazi Germany, the Nuremberg Code forbade forced medical procedures, and the Helsinki Code is equally explicit that all patients have the right to informed consent before submitting to them. There's no informed consent for vaccine mandates.[5]

In a workshop on vaccines, Larry Palevsky, MD, another board-certified pediatrician opposing the mandates, explores the very same themes:

> I was taught that vaccines were completely safe and effective, and for years I used them. But my experience, and what parents and doctors were telling me, was that vaccines aren't completely safe or effective. We were taught that polio, smallpox, and most infectious diseases went away because of vaccines. But the literature shows that diphtheria, tetanus, polio, pertussis, measles, influenza, TB, and scarlet fever were already waning before antibiotics and vaccines, because of clean water, better living conditions, sanitation, and nutrition. Other studies show that antibodies aren't how the body is protected, and that some vaccines contain foreign DNA that accumulates in the body and brain, and impairs the immune system. What we have now is a one-sided way of thinking that doesn't allow debate.
>
> It's heartbreaking to see kids who were speaking, doing well, and developmentally normal, who lost their voice, made no eye contact, developed seizures, asthma, and allergies, and had nowhere to go because the doctor said it was a coincidence. The studies that deny any correlation between vaccination and autism don't meet scientific standards.[6]

While theirs are some of the most familiar voices, I could go on and on; as more and more vaccines are introduced and mandated, the roster of family doctors, pediatricians, and other doctors speaking out against mandatory vaccinations and questioning the official dogma surrounding them grows larger by the day. No matter where and in what manner they practice, or what their specialty, their arguments and objections are all remarkably similar, invoking and elaborating on the very same themes that Dr. Mendelsohn presciently identified a generation ago. Rather than opposing all vaccines across the board, they favor a pro-choice position, as I do: they want safer vaccines, expose cover-ups, demand full disclosure by the industry and the CDC, insist on informed consent, and oppose making vaccination mandatory.

And hiding behind them stand many more who feel the same way but are afraid to say so openly. In one study that interviewed general pediatricians and pediatric subspecialists, 10% of the former and 21% of the latter admitted that they would not follow the CDC mandates in vaccinating their own children in the future;[7] many planned to postpone the MMR at least until after 18 months of age, and to reject the rotavirus, meningococcus, and hepatitis A vaccines altogether.[8]

WHAT PARENTS KNOW FOR SURE

The other side of the equation, and the larger and weightier truth that an important part of our job involves simply bearing witness to, encompasses thousands upon thousands of stories of vaccine-injured kids and the parents, relatives, and friends who care for and about them. I recently came across a questionnaire devised by Larry Cook, an activist on behalf of the vaccine-injured, and cofounder of StopMandatoryVaccinations.com, which he posted on Facebook as a vehicle for collecting as many personal narratives as possible:

> How did you decide to start researching vaccine safety and efficacy?
> What was the defining moment that convinced you not to vaccinate?
> Was it a person or personal relationship, or an educational material (book, article, video, etc.) that started you on this path of investigation?
> Have you ever regretted not vaccinating, and if so, why?[9]

What follows is a small sampling of the hundreds of replies that he has received so far, chosen to reflect the broad diversity of their personal histories and motives, and the lifelike quality of their personal narratives, to reaffirm the accuracy and validity of the clinical perspective:

Lifelong Guilt

"My son died 40 hours after his 2-month shots. I'd never heard of vaccine injury before. I feel guilty every day because it was the one thing I didn't look into and wish I did."

Coercion

"I work for the state, and the insurance is fantastic; but I have to follow their 'health enhancement program,' doing physicals, well visits, and things like that. They say it's a choice; but if you choose not to, the cost triples and I can't afford that. Luckily our pediatrician doesn't force the issue. But if childhood vaccines became compulsory, I'd have to drop the insurance, and we'd be screwed."

Telling Lies

"I'm a nurse and gave the flu vaccine to employees. We were not supposed to get vaccine on our hands. We also had to tell pregnant women the preservative-free shot has no mercury. But it does, and it makes everyone sick. The company I worked for told us we had to tell them it was a coincidence."

Medical Inattention

"My daughter had a severe reaction to her 18-month shots, and we nearly lost her. I reported it, but they didn't bat an eye! That's when I started researching! It was a huge wake-up call. No one in my family will ever vaccinate again!"

Nervous System Dysfunction, and More

"Behavior changes to my four-year-old after her MMR-II and DTaP-IPV are what did it. Eczema, sleep disorder, glassy eyes, drooling, and anger. She wasn't herself, and the only difference was the vaccines."

Autism

"Hours after my son's 12-month check-up, I remember looking back at him in the car; his eyes were rolling back into his head, and he was spitting up in an unusual way. I screamed and drove to the ER like a mad woman. He was hospitalized for three days with a temp of 105.7°. When the nurses put tubes in his head to drain the swelling, they told me to calm down because vaccine reactions like this were normal; but what's normal about that? And then I vaccinated him again! I just did what I was told.

"But after that, I started reading, and found out that what he went through wasn't normal; and he hasn't been vaccinated since. At age five, my beautiful son was diagnosed with Autism Spectrum; it had taken three and a half years before anyone would listen to me. My six-year-old has never been vaccinated. People don't understand my passion about this."

Bearing Witness

"I worked in a doctor's office and saw so many people coming in extremely sick after receiving their flu shots! That raised some red flags, as did noticing how carelessly the medical practices were handled, like the drugs brought in by the sales reps who bought us lunch and handed them out like candy. That started me doubting, and when I got pregnant I began doubting the vaccines too. After extensive research and talking with many parents on both sides of the issue, I was sure that vaccines aren't for us!"

Family History

"When my son was two, he was vaccinated, became lethargic, went into respiratory distress, and was hospitalized for over two months. They said it was one in a million, and would never happen again. We continued vaccinating him on a delayed schedule, but he continued to get sicker; and still I was reassured by the doctors that we were doing the right thing. My son is now going on six, and our daughter is 18 months, also vaccinated on a delayed schedule. She gets extreme fevers, goes lethargic, and 'zones out'; again they tell us, it's 'just so rare!' We held off on giving her more; but she still wasn't meeting her milestones, and developed serious GI problems. At this point we stopped vaccinating, and started researching.

"Our two youngest aren't vaccinated at all and are never sick, while our two oldest are chronically ill to this day. I too had severe reactions to a flu shot in 1997 and my second Hep B in 1999. With our family history of psoriasis, eczema, and autoimmune diseases, we should never have been vaccinated in the first place!"

An Array of Symptoms

"I kept trying to figure out how my two-year-old had become so ill. Reading his medical records reminded me that he'd had a reaction for up to ten days after each vaccination, anything from a rash to hives, fever, or screaming oddly for hours at a time, but all worrisome enough that we took him to the ER each time. It's taken years to restore his health, to the point that we've stopped vaccinating all our children."

Asthma, Allergies, Asperger's

"In 1980, I vaccinated my first child as instructed; there were a few issues, but I didn't connect them. In 1985, with our second, I'd read about problems with some vaccines, so we did the DT only; still she developed chronic asthma and allergies. But our third developed Asperger's from his vaccines. By then there were many more on the schedule; thank God we didn't do them all! He has suffered the most, after receiving the MMR three times in his teens, and the chicken pox, both of which I approved of at the time. Now we're spending thousands to try to restore his health: he's very ill."

Brain Damage

"I witnessed my friend's daughter having an adverse reaction to the HPV vaccine at 18 years of age. The day after being vaccinated, she had a stroke, spent over a month in the hospital, had to relearn how to talk and walk again, and lost much of her memory. Four years later, she is still recovering."

ADHD and Autism

"After being vaccinated, my baby regressed, screamed for days, and became sick with multiple ear infections, despite being 100% breastfed. He now has ADHD and Autism-Spectrum issues. Against my better judgment, I was also pressured into a flu shot when I was eight months pregnant with him. My unvaccinated children have not suffered anything like that. Knowing what I know now and wish I'd known then, I'll never vaccinate another baby."

Bullied

"My son was injured from a vaccine, and his injuries were bad; but it wasn't until I was also injured by the same vaccine that I fully comprehended how bad it was. Crawling on all fours to look after my children was my light-bulb moment. Right then we moved away from mainstream medicine, but I still regret that I allowed myself to be bullied into vaccinating my children, and that the doctors refused to acknowledge my fears and concerns. From that day on, I would've stepped in front of a bullet to spare my children any further damage. My third child was born at home 24 years ago, with no vitamin K or eye drops; she has never been vaccinated, is the healthiest of my three, and the only one with higher education beyond high school. She has two degrees, including a Master's in Education; my other two are both disabled."

Her Pet Dog

"My prized English bulldog went into anaphylactic shock after her third booster shot! That's what got me started asking vets about vaccines; and they gave me no clear answers! That's how I came across so much information. After seeing my dog so close to death and realizing this could happen to my children, I decided I wasn't willing to take the risk!"

Family History

"In my teens, my mom told me that an uncle just died from the swine flu shot, and that I ran 106° fevers twice and nearly died after being vaccinated as a baby in the late fifties. Then she added that our cousin developed a mental condition that they didn't have a name for then, but probably was autism, and the whole family believed it was the vaccines that did it, because he changed right after that. Right then, I thought, there's got to be something fishy about this vaccinating thing. Growing up in Sacramento in the seventies, I knew many people who didn't vaccinate, and started talking to Preventive Medicine doctors and local health gurus. I decided not to vaccinate long before I was married and had my daughter in 1982."

The Medical System

"I almost died from being given prescription drugs for a month and a half, followed by others for a whole year, during which time I suffered so much in so many ways that I ended up firing my doctors, and told them I'd decided to find my own natural cure. It took me a couple of years of nonstop reading, but I succeeded. After that, I started researching foods, beauty products, vaccines, everything!"

Past Medical History

"It took me falling ill after hospital-mandated flu and H1N1 vaccines. My son almost died the day after his two-month shots, but I believed the docs, who ruled it an 'acute, life-threatening episode of SIDS,' in spite of the fact that he didn't die. He became seriously ill again after his Seventh-Grade series, at about the same time that I got sick from mine. With him, I didn't notice it immediately; the doctor said he was just going through puberty, and this and that. It wasn't until six months later that his pediatrician took our complaints seriously and discovered that he had a brain tumor."

Overkill

"I was an ignorant mom who followed my pediatrician's advice. My gut made me ask questions, and I had the sense to spread out the vaccines and not do multiple cocktails. But each time, my kids got fevers, welts, and felt crummy, while I lost a lot of sleep worrying about them. Still it wasn't till the flu shots made my kids really sick that I said, 'No More!' Even so, they keep pushing whooping cough and HPV, and we keep refusing them. I did my research and chose to stop vaccinating when my children were in Third and Fourth Grade. Now they both have Personal-Belief Exemptions and won't get any more shots; I haven't had any more either."

A Parent's Intuition

"It was an innate, clear understanding that vaccines weren't safe or effective and represented a clear and present danger. It was something I knew instinctively, and nothing done or said to me could alter it; in fact, every insult and embarrassment I suffered because of it only strengthened that resolve."

Ditto

"I just had a feeling: I knew that if anything happened to my daughter as a result of a vaccination, I'd never forgive myself."

A Nurse's Doubts

"I'm an RN working in the NICU for 27 years. When we started vaccinating babies less than an hour old for Hep B, it didn't seem right; these are newborns with no risk factors, whose moms tested negative for Hep B. When I asked about it, I was told to do it anyway, 'because it's the law.' Soon after, flu vaccines were mandated for us, though I'd never had one in my life; and that triggered my research, and my discovery of corruption and greed in the vaccine establishment."

A Teacher's Fears

"I'm a teacher; two different moms told me of their perfectly normal children who regressed into autism immediately after vaccines."

Death

"In 1981 my son suffered severe reactions to DPT vaccines at 8 and 13 months; he should never have received the second, which resulted in encephalitis, with high fever and vomiting, after which his health deteriorated; at the age of two, he finally slipped away."

A Bad Case of Denial

"My son got the MMR. Two weeks later he complained that his heart was racing; the rate was 160 per minute, but it went back to normal in a minute or so. The cardiologist did a lot of tests and sent us home with a heart monitor to put on when his heart raced; but he reassured me that the MMR didn't cause it. Blindly I just did what I was told; 6 months later he died from supraventricular tachycardia.

"Two years later, when Jared was three and Seth nine months, Jared got the MMR, and Seth got DTaP, Hib, and polio. Seth cried for two hours afterward, and stopped walking, started banging his head, and didn't speak for two years. I can't convey how desperate I felt watching another son deteriorate right in front of me and feeling helpless to stop it. At 18 months he was diagnosed as severely autistic, and once again I was told it wasn't the shots, that it was 'just a coincidence' and was going to happen no matter what.

"Meanwhile, nine days after his MMR, Jared started seizing, and again I was told it was a coincidence, not the MMR. Still I went along; but after three months, Seth went in for another round, and the girl who checked us in gave me vaccine information sheets, which shocked me, because no one had ever given them to me before; I didn't even know they existed! On the MMR sheet I read that 6 in 10,000 children suffer seizures, brain damage or death! WTF, when my pediatrician walked in, I lost my fucking religion! Needless to say, no shots were given that day! That's when I finally started doing my own research, logging onto *Pub Med, Postgraduate Medicine,* the CDC website, and the package inserts; I couldn't believe what I was reading; everything I'd been taught was a lie."

"Natural Causes"

"My son died and my daughter was injured after their vaccinations. The Coroner told me that my son died of 'natural causes,' namely, SIDS. My daughter's injury was labeled 'coincidental.' The Coroner warned me not to mention vaccines as a possible cause of my son's death, or I'd be charged with contempt of court. *They know.*"[10]

As their stories make clear, these parents, relatives, eyewitnesses, victims, and friends are not antiscientific zealots wedded to a fixed ideological position, but simply people whose lives and perspectives have been turned upside down, and in many cases ruined, by what happened to them or their children, friends, and loved ones.

SOME VACCINE CASES OF MY OWN

In much the same way, my own patients' histories have taught me that the committed relationships, memorable experiences, and the commonsense reasoning involved in raising a child provide a far more accurate context for determining whether a vaccine has played a causal or contributory role in the problems that follow it than any preformed list of "acceptable" or "proven" reactions. If applied in good faith with an open mind, facilitated if necessary by a caring physician or health professional, the parental instinct is well adapted to figuring out what really happened and why, without the necessity for an elaborate, quasi-judicial procedure.

On the other hand, as I will presently show, even intelligent, attentive parents can easily miss the vaccine connection in the case of chronic, autoimmune diseases, which often require months or even years to develop, and may not become manifest even then without another insult, such as a booster shot or exposure to toxic chemicals.

To illustrate, here is the tale of a twelve-year-old boy whom I know of solely from his mother's letter, but her words are so heartfelt and so congruent with the whole of my experience that I cannot imagine them to be anything but the honest truth as she experienced it; and I venture to say that even my most obdurate critics will be hard put to reject them out of hand:

> My son Adam was healthy until his first MMR at 15 months. Within two weeks he had flu and cold symptoms that persisted for six weeks, at which point his eyes had become puffy, and he was hospitalized with nephrotic syndrome. A renal biopsy showed "focal sclerosing glomerulonephritis," but he didn't respond to steroids. I asked if it could be related to the vaccine, but they told me it couldn't, and we accepted that.
>
> Over the next four years he was hospitalized repeatedly, but finally went into remission, seeming normal and healthy, and stayed off all medication for five years. When he turned 10, his pediatrician recommended a booster, saying that a rise in measles cases made it dangerous for him not to be protected. Checking the *PDR* and other sources, I found no warning for kidney disease or listing of it as an adverse reaction; so I agreed to it. In less than two weeks, he relapsed, with ++++ protein in the urine, swelling, and massive weight gain, signs that we recognized at once. He was admitted in hypertensive crisis, with blood in the urine, fluid in the lungs, and generalized edema. On Cytoxan, massive doses of Prednisone, and three other drugs he slowly improved, but missed another seven months of school.
>
> It's been two years since that horrible episode, and he still needs Captopril for high blood pressure and spills ++++ protein every day. The doctor says he sustained major kidney damage, will always need medication to control his blood pressure, and will worsen as he grows, necessitating a transplant eventually. This time I was convinced that his condition was related to the vaccine, but still the doctors didn't take me seriously and told me it was a coincidence.
>
> I searched for information and even contacted the manufacturer of the vaccine. Finally they sent me two almost identical reports of nephrotic syndrome following the MMR vaccine. It's very difficult for lay people to get information or even ask questions, since we don't use correct medical terms and feel stupid. Please tell me if my ideas are reasonable. I don't think my son could tolerate another episode, and I think he'd have normal blood pressure and kidney function today if not for that second shot.
>
> I also have great concern for other children who develop nephrotic syndrome some weeks after receiving MMR and whose doctors never make the connection. They could all be at great risk if revaccinated. I realize that this letter has taken up a lot of your time, and I'd appreciate any help you can give me. Thank you.[11]

Like many others who seek my help, this woman honestly believed that the MMR vaccine had crippled her son for life; yet she had no intention of suing the drug company who manufactured it, the doctors who administered it, or the government's Vaccine Injury Compensation Program, as she was legally entitled to do. Whether she didn't think she could win, a conclusion my experience would certainly justify, or just wasn't a litigious person, as seems more relevant in her case, the absence of such motive only lends further credence to her story. She was writing simply to find a physician to hear and validate the truth of her experience, which neither the pediatrician who recommended and gave the shots, nor the specialists who treated Adam in the hospital, nor any of the other doctors she spoke to were willing to do. Although it was very little to ask, it was more than enough to earn her gratitude.

To anyone inclined to discredit such tales, I need only repeat that the confidences our patients entrust to us represent the truth as they live it, and that in this instance the causal link between the vaccine and the disease that ruined Adam's life is sufficiently obvious to be grasped at once by any reasonably attentive twelve-year-old of average intelligence. Yet when vaccines are involved, such stories are routinely dismissed out of hand, by parents and doctors alike, as if they couldn't possibly be true or worthy of serious consideration, or at most a rare event, tragic to be sure, but of no statistical significance.

Even in the face of compelling circumstantial evidence to the contrary, "a coincidence" was the automatic response of every doctor involved in Adam's care, and they stuck to it even when two virtually identical case reports were supplied by the drug company itself. Whether a canny strategy to defeat possible litigation, or simply the instinctive shielding of a cherished worldview from the threat of change, this prejudice is so deeply ingrained in the medical profession as to warrant careful study in itself.

Finally, Adam's by no means unique misfortune calls further attention to the largely unexamined deliberations as to whether or not "glomerulonephritis," "autism," "encephalopathy," or any other such complication is judged to have been caused by a vaccine or vaccines and thus qualifies as legally compensable. As for Adam in particular, notwithstanding the two cases of MMR nephritis documented by the manufacturer, renal failure is still not officially recognized as an adverse effect of the vaccine, an omission that not only helped the doctors to frustrate his mother's inquiries, but would undoubtedly have assured her defeat in the VICP "court" had she chosen that route.

In short, even though the complication it describes is too uncommon to qualify as a smoking gun in the statistical sense, this case illustrates all of the issues we have just been discussing, and also foreshadows the chapters to follow. I can imagine no more powerful indictment of the VICP, our current program for compensating vaccine-injured patients, than its deafness to tragedies as transparent and heartrending as this one.

EAR INFECTIONS: MAKING WORSE WHAT'S ALREADY THERE

Relatively few of the vaccine-related complications I have witnessed in my own patients have been as severe as Adam's; for the most part, they seem to indicate another, more generic level of vaccine involvement that is common enough to be the rule rather than the exception, and may thus indicate how vaccines appear to act in most people, even when there is no obvious, flagrant, or immediate ailment to show for it.

At first, the only vaccine reactions I was sure of were relatively minor illnesses that I traced to a specific vaccine component because of symptoms that were highly suggestive of the corresponding disease, such as inflamed, painful parotids and swollen retroauricular and suboccipital lymph nodes from the mumps and rubella components of the MMR, or a fever of 105° and a blood smear featuring a white blood cell count of 32,000 per cu mm after the DPT, including 20% immature band forms, and 1% metamyelocytes and other still more immature forms, which a pediatrician friend looked at and immediately identified as pertussis.[12]

As the years went by, with more and more vaccines being mandated, and often several being given at once, it became increasingly difficult to isolate a specific vaccine or component as solely responsible; but I began to notice that children recently vaccinated seemed to react nonspecifically by becoming especially prone to contract whatever acute illnesses were going around their school or neighborhood, or to develop a more intense or chronic version of whatever illnesses they were already bothered by, such as ear infections, which were virtually ubiquitous at that time.

In this typical example, a nineteen-month-old girl came down with a series of ear infections after her MMR vaccine, together with a bad flare-up of eczema and nasal allergies, both of which she had had only mildly since her birth:

> Already a veteran of five ear infections and as many rounds of antibiotics since her MMR vaccine at 15 months, a 19-month-old girl also developed severe eczema and nasal allergies over the same period. Although these latter

> complaints began in early infancy, they had remained quite mild, with the eczema confined to a few small patches on the face and behind the ears.
>
> With no overt reaction to her DPT's, she developed her first ear infection with fever shortly after weaning and entering day care around her first birthday. After that she seemed fine until her MMR, soon after which her ears flared up repeatedly, with high fever, earache, and listless, clingy behavior, and never wholly cleared up, despite five rounds of antibiotics. Meanwhile, her allergies became severe and unrelenting, and the eczema spread over her whole body.
>
> After the parents decided not to vaccinate her temporarily, her ears cleared up nicely. Now twelve, she has normal hearing, and has remained in good health otherwise; but her parents remain dead set against resuming her shots.[13]

In this case, while the girl was clearly affected by the MMR more than the DPT, her reaction was limited to recurrent ear infections and an intensification of the eczema and nasal allergies she had had before. Since all three ailments number among the commonest illnesses of her age group, her mother never suspected vaccines until a stretch of uninterrupted good health abruptly came to an end soon after giving her one.

The possibility that otitis media might be a specific reaction to the MMR was ruled out by this case of recurrent ear infections in a six-year-old girl, culminating in a particularly severe episode after her DPT booster before entering first grade:

> Beginning at five months of age, the episodes were characterized by red cheeks, grumpy and irritable behavior, and loss of appetite, but rarely fever or earache. Afterwards, she typically complained of runny, itchy eyes, and seemed generally "run down," needing more sleep, and more likely to catch whatever her friends and relatives were bringing over, which the mother wearily described as "being sick all the time."
>
> She had had all her shots, which in those days consisted only of DPT and polio at 2, 4, 6, and 18 months, one MMR at 15 months, and a final DPT before first grade. Although the ear infections had continued at frequent intervals, the last booster brought on an unusually severe episode that lasted for 4 months without a break, in spite of the antibiotics, and finally persuaded her mother to try a different approach.
>
> Several months after holistic treatment and putting off any further shots, the mother phoned to say that the ear infections were gone, and the occasional

> colds and acute illnesses were quickly disposed of. Three years later, she reported that her daughter hadn't missed a single day of school, and was thriving in every way.[14]

Acute and Chronic

From a large number of similar ear infection cases, I began to understand that these children were reacting to something inherent in the vaccination process itself, rather than to any particular vaccine, because it seemed that any vaccine might suffice, and its main effect was either to activate whatever disease tendencies might be latent in that particular child, or to exacerbate and make more chronic the ones that were already manifest, including but by no means limited to the broad spectrum of diseases most prevalent in that age group.

An instructive variation on the general theme was this story of a toddler who had already lived through eleven ear infections and as many rounds of antibiotics by the time I first saw her:

> Otherwise in good health, a chubby girl of 15 months was brought in for repeated ear infections, which had never cleared up despite eleven rounds of antibiotics. After a good pregnancy and easy labor, her mother chose not to nurse, and the child developed her first ear infection, with a fever of 103° and violent earache, at two months of age, soon after her first DPT, Hib, and polio combination.
>
> All later episodes were afebrile, typically with fretting and pulling at the ear; and twice she was treated with antibiotics at a regular checkup, with no symptoms at all, just because the pediatrician had detected some fluid behind the drum.
>
> Not long after her parents voted for holistic treatment and decided to stop vaccinating her for a while, the girl became acutely ill, with a high fever and loud screaming, a virtual replica of her original attack, from which she recovered in less than a day. She never had another episode. By her next visit, three months later, she was completely well and thriving in every way. That was over three years ago, and since that time she has had no ear infections, no antibiotics, and, at her parents' insistence, no more shots.[15]

In this case, the only clear link to any vaccine was her first episode, which followed her first series of vaccines at two months, after which her condition became so chronic that the later doses made no apparent difference. What especially interested me was her last episode, which was acute and violent, with fever and intense pain, just like her first one, and resulted in complete recovery. From it and many others like it, I have learned to regard most acute illnesses with fever and strong, well-marked symptoms as generally favorable prognostic signs, indicating strong vitality and an immune system that is developing normally, and to worry more about children who seem unable to mount fevers and other acute responses to infection, as the healthy immune system seems "hardwired" to do.

So often forgotten or lost sight of, this obvious and fundamental lesson helped me realize that, over and above their intended effect of producing specific antibodies to the virus or bacterium in question, vaccines also, by some mechanism as yet undetermined, bring about the unintended and undesirable result of reprogramming the child's developing immune system to respond more chronically and less acutely in general (i.e., *nonspecifically*), whichever vaccine is given, and no matter what the illness that follows it.

ANY VACCINE WILL DO

As if to underline the point, here is the case of a little girl who developed a nearly identical pattern of ear infections following two different vaccines:

> A baby girl of ten months was brought in for otitis media, with high fever, intense earache, and loud screaming, her fifth such episode since two months of age, each one beginning soon after finishing the antibiotic from the one before. Even before that, as a newborn, she became fussy when her mother weaned her to go back to work, and developed a florid rash from her milk-based formula.
>
> All of these symptoms were intensified soon after her first DPT, Hib, and oral polio combination, culminating in her first ear infection two weeks later, with high fever and violent earache. After that she received only the DT, and had no overt reaction to it at all; but her ear infections continued unabated, as before.
>
> When her mother began holistic treatment and declared a moratorium on vaccines and antibiotics, they quickly subsided. But they came back with a vengeance six months later, when her parents separated, and her father insisted on taking her for the MMR, followed by three typical ear infections and as many rounds of antibiotics in rapid succession.

> Once again, she recovered well under her mother's care and remained in very good health overall, in spite of a tendency to relapse when she visited her father, who indulged her with dairy products and took her to the doctor for her full quota of vaccines and antibiotics. Now a freshman in college, she still gets sick at times, but her ear infections are long gone, and her immune system responds acutely and vigorously each time, with prompt, long-lasting recovery.[16]

This girl's almost identical reaction to two different vaccine combinations indicated a definite predisposition to fall ill in a certain way that was recognizably her own, and most likely already in place to some extent even before the vaccines were given; their obvious and important contribution being simply to reactivate and exacerbate it, and ultimately to establish it as a chronic pattern.

According to industry protocols and CDC standards, this preexisting susceptibility would disqualify such a case from being counted as vaccine-related, and would therefore all but assure her defeat if it resulted in a claim for damages in the VICP court. This conceptual road not taken could also help explain why so few scientists have thought to investigate any possible downside of the vaccination process *per se*; yet simply looking at this case through the magnifying lens of the clinical perspective makes clear why they should.

NONSPECIFIC REACTIONS THE RULE, NOT THE EXCEPTION

Here is the simplest possible illustration of the same phenomenon, involving a teenage girl whose distinctive ensemble of childhood complaints resurfaced after more than ten years within a week of being given an MMR booster as a requirement for entering college:

> A patient of mine since childhood, an 18-year-old girl was preparing to leave for college. In primary school, she had suffered a great deal from enuresis and an obsessive-compulsive tendency, but had successfully overcome these symptoms, and with the help of holistic medicine had remained largely symptom-free for more than ten years. Within a week after her MMR booster, her old pattern of bedwetting and OCD behaviors returned in full force. Fortunately, she again recovered promptly, and has remained well since.[17]

In like manner, most of the adverse effects of vaccines that I have witnessed in my own patients represent a wide variety of nonspecific reactions to vaccination, and take the form of an easily recognizable pattern of the patient, rather than a statistically significant effect of any particular vaccine. By no means necessarily minor or trivial, they encompass the same broad spectrum of ailments seen in every general pediatric practice, including asthma, eczema, sinusitis, allergies, ADHD, learning and behavior problems, autism, and so forth.

Here follows the tale of a young boy with croup and mental retardation, born to a diabetic mother and already significantly handicapped at birth, yet clearly pushed into a steep decline by his vaccines. He was brought back with some difficulty to a reasonable state of health, and then suffered a still more profound relapse from a long-delayed second round:

> A 15-month-old boy was brought in for croup, recurrent colds, and developmental issues. Born to a diabetic mother, he weighed 8 pounds at birth and spent weeks on a respirator in the Newborn ICU for "undeveloped lungs," with cyanosis and unstable blood sugars. In the early months he was colicky and had a severe diarrhea that stopped when his mother eliminated wheat from her diet.
>
> At three months, soon after his first DPT, Hib, and OPV combination, he became very restless, with swollen glands and a sickly pallor that lasted for months, and culminated in a prolonged attack of croup, high fever, and sunken chest that required hospitalization and IV corticosteroids for relief. When the cough persisted, his mother put off the second round of shots for many months, but the same croupy cough came right back after she finally agreed to it, as did the swollen glands and exactly the same symptoms as before.
>
> With a marked fear of strangers, the boy appeared subnormal when I first saw him, drooling profusely, with his mouth hanging open, and hiding behind his mother. Fortunately, with the help of natural remedies, and no vaccines, antibiotics, or steroids, his illness cleared up; and a month later his mother was ecstatic, with no croup and no swollen glands in the dead of winter. That was six years ago, and I've not seen them since; but his mother called recently to report that he is still "thriving and developing normally, like other children his age."[18]

Another boy with severe, year-round asthma achieved a sustained improvement with holistic care, but relapsed almost immediately after a DPT booster:

> Asthmatic since the age of two, and testing positive for a broad spectrum of allergens, a four-year-old boy was brought in because even a daily regime of bronchodilators and inhaled corticosteroids had not prevented major flare-ups

the previous fall and winter, several of them requiring oral prednisone and antibiotics as well. Within a few months of beginning holistic treatment, he had cut his inhaled steroids by half, maintained higher peak flows of 150 or more, and even recovered from a cold without developing asthma or requiring any drugs for the first time in his life.

The following spring and summer, at the peak of his allergy season, he was still doing well on half-doses of his inhaler, and remained healthy and energetic, with average peak flows at record levels of 160–175. That fall he got his DPT booster before entering kindergarten, promptly came down with bronchitis, and his allergies returned in full force. Once again, he responded well to stopping the drugs and vaccines, and has continued to improve over the past two years, without needing to resume them.[19]

Another example was this girl with a seizure disorder, first appearing in infancy, which her parents had no doubt was caused by a round of vaccinations, but continued to worsen even after they stopped vaccinating her, and reached its full intensity only a year later:

A three-year-old girl was brought in to see me for frequent attacks of "shuddering," in which she tensed her limbs, shook her head, and stiffened her body. Although the pregnancy was complicated by first-trimester bleeding, exposure to toxic chemicals, and IV antibiotics during labor for a Group B Strep infection, the child appeared perfectly healthy at birth, nursed well, and remained alert and energetic for the first two months of her life.

Upon receiving her first DPT, Hib, and oral polio combination, she screamed violently for three days and began spitting up excessively after feedings, a pattern that cleared up, but then reappeared with teething. At six months, the shuddering episodes began, shortly after her third round of vaccines, which convinced her parents to stop vaccinating her for good. Sporadic and intermittent at first, they grew steadily more frequent when solid foods were introduced. By her second birthday, they were occurring around 200 times a day on average, with arms extended and thumbs tucked into her palms.

Although she was intelligent and highly verbal, her mental development had also been adversely affected by the seizures, which were especially frequent after milk and dairy. Gentle and sweet-natured for the most part, she was prone to unpredictable outbursts of violent temper at times when her attacks were especially frequent, with screaming, biting, and a predilection for smashing things. She was also quite afraid of loud noises, and of bedtime and going to sleep.

After postponing any further vaccines or medications, and beginning a more holistic approach, her parents noted a definite improvement in her mood and energy; and gradually her seizures became fewer, briefer, less intense, and less easily provoked, while her mood, energy, and speech also improved, with fewer angry outbursts. Within three months the attacks had almost disappeared, and after six months she seemed an altogether different child, active and vivacious, as well as calmer and less troubled, and had made great leaps forward in speech and learning. Over the years since then, she has continued to thrive, with no shuddering, no tantrums, and no major reactions to occasional dairy treats; but her parents still refuse to consider revaccinating her.[20]

I present these cases to call attention to what appears to be a nonspecific effect of all vaccinations on the overall health of their recipients, namely, their tendency to add to or amplify whatever risks or predispositions to chronic disease are already present, even if the recipients don't become overtly ill at the time, but only predisposed to react more and more forcibly in the future, whether to subsequent vaccinations, or when exposed to drugs, chemicals, and allergens that they have become sensitized to as a result.

It seems clear that this sensitization also provides a missing link to the mounting toll of deaths and crippling, irreversible complications that we read about in the newspapers and the blogosphere, which are nevertheless still generally dismissed as unrelated.

As we shall see, this hypothesis is also strongly supported by current research on autoimmune phenomena, and also helps explain why adverse reactions to vaccines are so commonly overlooked and underreported, even by parents, and are sometimes difficult to recognize even when they are looked for.

1. They often don't manifest until many weeks or months after the shot, an interval well beyond the limit of most of those officially accepted and listed as such.
2. They involve a nonspecific reaction to the vaccination process *per se,* which few physicians seem interested in and few parents know to look for, rather than or in addition to a specific reaction to a specific vaccine.
3. They often involve activation of disease tendencies that were already latent in the particular child, or reactivation, exacerbation, or

progression into a chronic state of illnesses already manifest, and thus characteristic of the patient, rather than of any particular vaccine.

4. They involve many of the same illnesses that unvaccinated children are also coming down with, encompassing the whole spectrum of pediatric practice, including ear infections, eczema, asthma, allergies, sinusitis, ADD, learning disabilities, autism, and so forth.
5. They are common enough to be the rule, rather than the exception.
6. Any vaccine can produce them, and the affected children tend to react in more or less the same way each time to whichever vaccine they are most sensitive to, and sometimes to two or more different vaccines.
7. Other environmental factors, such as drugs, herbicides, pesticides, toxins, and pollutants are also frequently implicated, so that neither vaccines nor hereditary predispositions are the only causal factor.
8. With so many vaccines being given, and so little time in between them, the parents often fail to recognize the connection until the child gets well and remains unvaccinated for a number of months, but then relapses in the same fashion soon after the next shot or booster is given.

Representing the full spectrum of pediatric practice, the cases cited above exemplify the synergy operating among inherited predispositions, latent tendencies, and vaccines in producing the illnesses we see in our offices, a collaboration that highlights the impossibility of attributing them exclusively to genetics or environment, the traditional dichotomy that pro-vaccine circles still cling to.

While perhaps accepting the validity of this or that individual case, some readers may object that the main issue with such "anecdotal evidence" is simply one of frequency, which hasn't been honestly investigated, as we saw, so that these few individual case reports cannot provide adequate justification for rejecting the whole program. To these skeptics I need only repeat that the automatic, instinctive, and almost unanimous resistance of pediatricians across the board to worrying about the risks of vaccinating at all, let alone of piling on as many vaccines as the traffic will bear, has surely had the effect of dismissing such anecdotes and thus making the real injuries seem much less common than they really are.

THE "SMOKING GUNS"

On the other hand, such relatively ordinary cases are even less likely to satisfy the parents of dead or severely vaccine-injured children, who understandably seek a level of brute force wielding the same degree of causal power that killed their sons and daughters or crippled them for life. To them, having been compelled to endure such grievous losses and catastrophic illnesses day after day for years on end, simply making worse what's already there seems far too weak, subtle, and tenuous a link to do justice to the physical and emotional shock of whatever has shattered their peace and contentment for quite probably the rest of their lives.

For their sake, it is necessary to take another look at the big picture, and to focus on the genuine "smoking guns" that are indeed out there and have been identified so far, the most grievous, terrible, and all-too-frequent outcomes that vaccines are capable of. But these worst cases cannot be properly understood without being mindful of the insidious and at first subclinical alterations that so often prepare the ground for them to manifest at a later date.

SUMMARY

The clinical encounter between a doctor and a patient remains the simplest and often the most practical setting for determining whether or not an adverse reaction is vaccine-related. This is borne out by the personal histories of doctors who have begun to question and doubt our official vaccination policies, and by those parents who have witnessed their children's vaccine injuries or who refuse to vaccinate based on their own independent research.

My own experience with vaccine-related morbidity began with relatively minor reactions to specific vaccines exhibiting anatomical or physiological features typical of the natural disease. Eventually I learned to recognize nonspecific reactions to the vaccination process in general, namely, ongoing chronic illnesses, such as recurrent ear infections, asthma, eczema, allergies, sinusitis, seizures, ADD, autism, learning disabilities, and indeed the whole spectrum of modern pediatrics, as more or less distinct from the rare acute, catastrophic events acknowledged by the VAERS system and made compensable under the VICP program.

These are accordingly more difficult to recognize, by parents and doctors alike, because they also involve exacerbation of preexisting tendencies that are characteristic of the individual, rather than of any specific vaccine; because they are common enough to be the rule rather than the exception and involve many of the same ailments that their unvaccinated classmates are also coming down with; and because they tend to develop more slowly and may not become symptomatic for months or even years beyond the CDC's narrow time limits.

The link to vaccination nevertheless becomes irrefutably clear when the children recover from their illnesses and are well for an extended period of time, but then relapse from a later or booster dose. The logical inference from these cases is that the vaccination process interferes with the basic immune function in everyone, whether they immediately become ill from it or not, such that they become increasingly sensitive to subsequent doses, and to other chemical, food, or environmental exposures. A significant number of highly sensitized individuals will then go on to develop serious and life-threatening complications, as we shall see.

Chapter 5

AUTOIMMUNE DISEASE

The next three chapters are devoted to serious, life-threatening illnesses and injuries that are common enough to represent major public health problems, and have been linked to vaccines by a solid body of established scientific evidence. As we've come to expect, they have been carefully and systematically hidden by the vaccine industry and its advocates to avoid being acknowledged as such, by a concerted strategy of flat-out denial, cover-up, and even the falsification of scientific data, as well as hiding the actual figures in a tangle of massive underreporting, studied ignorance, and simple lack of curiosity.

THE AUTOIMMUNE HYPOTHESIS

In chapter 1, I proposed the hypothesis that autoimmune mechanisms are built into the vaccination process, as the basic pathway by which all vaccines act to bring about their intended result in everyone, as well as the whole spectrum of adverse effects, both of which represent their true and still largely hidden cost. In this chapter, I will reconsider in more detail what is now known about the causal link between vaccinations and autoimmunity.

AUTOIMMUNE DISEASES APPEARING AFTER VACCINATION

As a first step, I will consider autoimmune diseases that have appeared promptly after vaccinations, and have been or should be causally linked to them. The first "smoking-gun" revelation of this type was provided by the gastroenterologist Dr. Andrew Wakefield, whose 1995 *Lancet* article showed that children vaccinated against the measles were much more likely to develop ulcerative colitis and Crohn's disease later in life than their unvaccinated controls, a finding that has been widely ignored but never refuted.[1]

What the vaccine industry felt so threatened by was his follow-up article three years later, which ignited a firestorm of vilification and character assassination and ended in his excommunication from the medical profession. But his license was revoked and his reputation destroyed solely on the basis of the allegation that he failed to inform the journal about his participation in a lawsuit on behalf of his subjects, not the still unchallenged evidence of his elegant biopsy specimens from the intestinal tracts of autistic children who had previously been given the MMR vaccine (namely, histologic changes in their lymphoid aggregations that closely resembled those of Crohn's disease and ulcerative colitis, both inflammatory bowel diseases of an autoimmune nature).[2]

Quite apart from subsequent virological studies that demonstrated specific antibodies to measles in these lesions, but not to mumps or rubella, these original findings already conclusively demonstrated an autoimmune mechanism in these autistic children, and have been duplicated by independent investigators in many different countries.[3] Over and above their shocking implication that the measles vaccine might indeed be a cause of autism—as many parents were already insisting—what his work proved beyond a doubt, and with much less fanfare, was that autism is an autoimmune disease that involves the gastrointestinal tract, crosses the blood-brain barrier, and possibly damages other organs and tissues as well, a linkage that is destined to change the course of medical history, and indeed has already done so.

THE SPECTRUM OF AUTOIMMUNE DISEASES CAUSED BY VACCINES

As a rough estimate, although grossly understated, to be sure, I compiled a list of the diseases so far identified as commonly or invariably autoimmune[4] and the mandated vaccines that even their package inserts admit may be causally linked to them:[5]

Disease	Vaccines
Guillain-Barré syndrome	DTaP, Hib, pneumo, varicella, Hep B, flu, MMR
Encephalopathy, encephalitis	DTaP, varicella, Hep B, MMR
Angionedema	DTaP, pneumo, rotavirus, varicella, flu
Urticaria	DTaP, pneumo, rotavirus, Hep B, flu, MMR
Thrombocytopenic purpura	DTaP, pneumo, varicella, Hep B, MMR
Henoch-Schönlein purpura	varicella, flu
Type 1 Diabetes (IDDM)	HPV, MMR
Lymphadenopathy	pneumo, Hep B, flu
Erythema nodosum	HPV, Hep B
Multiple sclerosis	HPV, Hep B
Optic neuritis	HPV, Hep B, MMR
Vasculitis	Hep B, Flu, MMR
Chronic fatigue syndrome	Hep B
Alopecia areata	Hep B
Systemic lupus (SLE)	Hep B
Glomerulonephritis	HPV
Hemolytic anemia	pneumo
Kawasaki syndrome	rotavirus
Aplastic anemia	varicella
Transverse myelitis	varicella
Pancreatitis	MMR

To these should be added the fast-growing list of other autoimmune diseases that have been linked to vaccines in the literature, but not yet included in the package inserts. Somewhat daunted by the Herculean labor of running them all down and matching them up in the same way, I chose as a representative example the hepatitis B vaccine, which has already added almost twenty other diseases to the list by itself, even as the CDC's Advisory Committee on Immunization Practices (ACIP) proudly hails it as one of the safest vaccines currently available:

> Hepatitis B vaccines are safe to administer to adults and children. More than 10,000,000 adults and 2,000,000 infants and children have been vaccinated in

> the US, and over 12,000,000 children worldwide. Pain at the injection site and fever have been among the most frequently reported side-effects, but no more so than in the controls receiving placebo or DPT. The incidence of anaphylaxis is low. Large-scale programs in Alaska, New Zealand, and Taiwan have not established an association with other adverse events.[6]

Although far from complete, and sometimes including only a single example of the given diagnosis, the following is a list of case reports of additional autoimmune diseases attributed to the Hep B vaccine in the literature:

Pericarditis[7]
Demyelinating polyneuropathy [8]
Cerebellar ataxia[9]
Bullous pemphigoid[10]
Lichen planus[11]
Dermatomyositis[12]
Reiter's syndrome[13]
Uveitis[14]
Retinal vein thrombosis[15]
Glomerulonephritis[16]
Demyelinating CNS diseases[17]
Aseptic meningitis[18]
Toxic granuloma[19]
Erythema multiforme[20]
Nephrotic syndrome[21]
Cryoglobulinemia[22]
Rheumatoid arthritis[23]
Thyroiditis[24]

Furthermore, it turns out that many diseases causally linked to vaccines but not yet proven to be autoimmune have also developed from taking other drugs, likewise suggesting the possibility of similar autoimmune dysfunctions mediated by antigen-antibody complexes, while still other diseases not yet linked to vaccines are being identified as autoimmune all the time. Indeed, autoimmune phenomena have been turning up whenever and wherever we've bothered to look for them, as if the term "autoimmune" were ultimately coextensive if not synonymous with chronicity itself, the still mysterious process whereby diseases manage to insinuate and establish themselves within the basic long-term physiology of patients.

In a recent commentary that appeared in the *British Medical Journal*, for example, biochemists from Japan, Italy, the Netherlands, and the United States reported on various inflammatory mechanisms of cellular immunity mediated by cytokines that have already been shown to be instrumental in the development and progression of atherosclerosis, no less.[25]

There are three main reasons why the relatively low incidence of any one particular disease should not be allowed to mislead us into minimizing the importance of the category. The first is the extensive underreporting of adverse vaccine reactions that has already been pointed out, based on overly restrictive guidelines, widespread mistrust in the fairness of the VICP process, and indeed the well-kept secret of its very existence.

Differences in Individual Susceptibility

The second reason is the obvious importance of preexisting genetic and epigenetic differences in susceptibility between individual patients, which help to determine the intensity of their reactions, as well as the organs and tissues specifically targeted, and are also regularly invoked to disqualify many vaccine reactions, as we saw, as if innate susceptibility and environmental "triggers" such as vaccines were mutually exclusive explanations.

Exactly analogous to the risk of unwanted side effects with any drug treatment, no matter how low the incidence of any particular complication may be, the aggregate total of all of them combined adds up to a very substantial risk that any given patient will suffer an adverse reaction of some kind, a kind of Russian roulette that our children are being made to play. This is the main concern of Dr. Yehuda Shoenfeld, perhaps the world's leading authority on autoimmune phenomena:

> The fact that vaccines are delivered to billions of people without preliminary screening for underlying susceptibility is of concern. It is naive to believe that all humans are alike. Autoimmune diseases have increasingly been recognized as having a genetic basis, mediated by HLA subtypes. For instance, celiac disease has been strongly associated with either of two haplotypes, MS with another, rheumatoid arthritis with two others, and type 1 diabetes with yet another. Thus certain genes create a genetic predisposition toward developing an autoimmune disease, and typically requiring some environmental trigger to evolve into a full-blown disease.[26]

Subclinical Autoimmunity and Chronicity

Especially in that last sentence, Dr. Shoenfeld also hints at a third reason—perhaps the most important of all—for not mistaking the absolute incidence figures of these various diseases following vaccination for the full extent of the problem, namely, that autoimmune reactions most often occur subclinically at first, such that autoantibodies against our own tissues are regularly detectable, even in the absence of clinically significant illness, or indeed of any signs and symptoms whatsoever:

> One such environmental trigger is viral or bacterial. Another may be the adjuvant mechanism. Adjuvants are substances which enhance the immune response and are routinely included in vaccine preparations, the most common of which are aluminum compounds. Although the activation of autoimmune mechanisms by adjuvants found in vaccines is common, the appearance of autoimmune disease is less so. Non-antigenic activation of the innate cellular immunity, as well as the expression of various regulatory cytokines, may determine if an autoimmune response remains limited and harmless or evolves into a full-blown disease.
>
> For example, it has been shown that the vaccine for Lyme disease is capable of triggering arthritis in genetically susceptible hamsters, and that, when the adjuvant aluminum hydroxide is added, 100 percent of the hamsters develop arthritis. The vaccine preservative Thimerosal has also been demonstrated to induce a systematic autoimmune syndrome in transgenic mice, while mice with a genetic susceptibility for autoimmune disease show profound behavioral and neuropathological disturbances.[27]

These subclinical autoimmune phenomena are especially important in explaining the fact that full-blown disease may develop very slowly over a period of months or years and not become manifest until long after the stringent ACIP guidelines would arbitrarily rule them out as vaccine-related (e.g., after another challenge, such as a subsequent dose).

THE ASIA SYNDROME

This realization accompanied the recent discovery of what Shoenfeld and his colleagues have named the ASIA syndrome:

We have recently reported a new syndrome, ASIA, the Autoimmune/inflammatory Syndrome Induced by Adjuvants, which encompasses a spectrum of immune-mediated diseases triggered by a stimulus such as silicone, aluminum, and other adjuvants, which have been found to induce autoimmune and inflammatory manifestations by themselves, both in animal models and in humans.

Although the ASIA syndrome may be labeled "new," it reflects old truths. In 1982, epidemiological, clinical, and animal research showed that Guillain-Barré syndrome and other demyelinating autoimmune neuropathies, such as acute disseminated encephalomyelitis and multiple sclerosis, could occur up to 10 months following vaccination.

In such cases, the disease would first manifest with vague symptoms, like arthralgias, myalgias, paresthesias, and weakness, which were frequently deemed insignificant and ignored by the treating physicians. These would progress slowly and insidiously until the patient was exposed to a secondary immune stimulus, an infection or vaccination, which would then trigger the acute disease. It was the secondary response that would bring about the overt manifestation of an already present but subclinical, long-term, persistent disease.

We recently described six cases of systemic lupus following HPV vaccination. In all six, two common features were observed, namely, a personal or familial susceptibility to autoimmunity and an adverse response to a previous dose of the vaccine. Similarly, an analysis of 93 cases of autoimmunity following Hep B vaccination identified two major susceptibility factors, 1) exacerbation of adverse symptoms following additional doses of the vaccine in 47%, and 2) a personal or familial history of autoimmunity in 21%.

Vaccines given to children and adults may contain whole weakened infectious agents, genetically engineered antigens of these, or synthetic peptides, as well as adjuvants, typically aluminum. In addition, they may contain diluents, preservatives (Thimerosal, formaldehyde), detergents (polysorbate 80), and residues of culture media (yeast, gelatin, bovine extract, monkey kidney cells, etc.). The safety of these residues has not been investigated, but some studies suggest that even trace amounts of them may not be safe.

What is obvious is that the typical vaccine contains all the necessary biochemical components to induce autoimmune manifestations. Physicians need to be aware that vaccinations can trigger serious, potentially disabling, and even fatal autoimmune manifestations in certain individuals. Given the fact that they are administered to previously healthy people, efforts should be made to identify those subjects who are more at risk. In addition, careful assessment should

> be made regarding further doses in those with histories of adverse reactions in the past. The necessity of multiple doses should also be considered, as the enhanced adjuvant effect heightens the risk. Finally, we encourage efforts to develop safer vaccines by the industry.[28]

Neurotoxic Reactions the Rule, Not the Exception

The discovery of the ASIA syndrome highlights the propensity of vaccine adjuvants such as aluminum salts to generate autoimmune complexes that easily cross the blood-brain barrier and result in various types of neuropathology and brain damage. When placed alongside the CDC's own skyrocketing figures for autism, which by 2014 was estimated to affect 1 in 45, or 2.22% of all children ages 3 to 17 in the United States,[29] as well as equally significant increases in Guillain-Barré syndrome, ADD, ADHD, and other serious post-vaccine neuropathies, we can begin to appreciate the scale of the epidemic of brain and nervous system diseases and disabilities that comprise the largest subgroup, if not the absolute majority, of all the autoimmune diseases that have likewise become rampant in this country in recent decades, and have never been satisfactorily explained.

The Role of Aluminum Adjuvants

Particularly since the discovery of the ASIA syndrome, most scientists interested in adverse reactions to vaccines have focused their attention on the role of adjuvants, especially aluminum. A leader in this field is Dr. Lucija Tomljenovic of the University of British Columbia, who found an article in the *Journal of the AMA* from 1911 that warned about the broad systemic toxicity of even the small amounts of aluminum salts present in baking powders and food preservatives:

> That the aluminum ion is very toxic is well known. That aluminized food yields soluble aluminum compounds to gastric juice has been demonstrated. That such soluble aluminum is in part absorbed and carried to other parts of the body by the blood can no longer be doubted. The facts in this paper will give emphasis to my conviction that aluminum should be excluded from food.[30]

Contemporary research by Tomljenovic, her colleague Christopher Shaw, and others has demonstrated that the brain and central nervous system bear the brunt of aluminum toxicity, regardless of whether the substance is ingested orally or injected in a vaccine,[31] and that the damage can manifest in a wide variety of neuropathic states, ranging from learning disabilities, memory loss, impaired concentration, and speech defects, to seizures, confusion, anxiety, repetitive behaviors, and insomnia.[32] Other studies have conclusively linked aluminum toxicity not only to Alzheimer's disease, but also to other forms of dementia, as well as Parkinson's disease, Lou Gehrig's disease (ALS), multiple sclerosis, autism, and the other types of neurological impairment seen in children, encompassing the whole spectrum of brain damage and neurological diseases commonly encountered today.[33]

The exact mechanisms for these effects are complex and will be considered in later chapters; but the discovery of the ASIA syndrome has clearly established that all of the various neurotoxicities of aluminum are mediated by a series of interrelated autoimmune mechanisms involving activation of macrophages, lymphocytes, and cytokines of the innate cellular system, and eventually of the antibody-producing plasma cells of the humoral system as well.[34]

Even more recently, the predilection of aluminum-containing vaccines for causing various forms of brain and central nervous system damage has been attributed in part to the remarkable ease with which nanoparticles of the aluminum adjuvants in vaccines are transported through the blood, across the blood-brain barrier, and into the brain and cerebrospinal fluid.[35] New evidence has emerged that also confirms what many have long suspected, that aluminum adjuvants can persist inside the human body for decades:

> The prolonged hyperactivation of the immune system and chronic inflammation triggered by the persistence of aluminum adjuvants inside the human body (for up to 11 years post-vaccination) are thought to be the principal factors underlying the toxicity of these compounds. One reason for this long retention is most likely its tight association with the vaccine antigen or other vaccine excipients—i.e., contaminant DNA. Even dietary aluminum has been shown to accumulate in the CNS over time, producing Alzheimer-like outcomes in experimental animals fed amounts equivalent to what humans consume through a typical Western diet.[36]

Finally, contrary to the argument of Dr. Offit and other pro-vaccine advocates that humans obtain much more aluminum from their diet and various cosmetics than from vaccines,[37] Tomljenovic and Shaw have pointed out that injecting vaccines directly into the muscle, bypassing the normal protective barriers of the skin and GI tract, is much more likely to result in toxic outcomes at much lower doses, since only 0.25% of dietary aluminum is absorbed systemically, and even that is rapidly filtered out by healthy kidneys, whereas the soluble injectable hydroxide, the commonest form, is absorbed into the blood almost entirely, and accumulates much more readily in the brain and various internal organs.[38]

SUMMARY

It is evident that many, if not all, adverse reactions to vaccines are mediated by autoimmune mechanisms, and that all vaccines are capable of producing them, either by means of viral nucleic acids attaching themselves directly to the host cell genome, as with the live-virus vaccines, or by the formation of antigen-antibody complexes mediated by aluminum and other adjuvants.

Individual differences in genetic and epigenetic susceptibility are important factors in determining which tissues and cell types are targeted, and to what extent. Autoimmune phenomena may be present subclinically and progress insidiously, without ever provoking signs and symptoms of overt disease, or perhaps do so only months or years later, after a subsequent vaccination or immunological challenge. Although many different organs and tissues may be involved, the central nervous system is almost always affected, and appears to play a crucial unifying role in most if not all of the pathologies that eventually develop and become manifest.

Finally, this research clearly documents an additional risk from administering a large number of vaccines simultaneously, and further strengthens the implication that the primary determinant of overall risk is the total vaccine load, the total number of individual vaccines or vaccine components administered over time, or in other words, the total exposure to the vaccination *process* in general, rather than to any particular vaccine.

What remains to be established is whether other common and likewise rapidly increasing chronic diseases of children, such as asthma, eczema, sinusitis, allergies, ear infections, and the like, are similarly mediated by autoimmune mechanisms in response to vaccinations, as my own clinical experience and that of many colleagues strongly suggests.

To decide this question will require investigating the extent to which autoimmune phenomena are detectable in healthy children, both vaccinated and otherwise, and thus widening the field beyond the brain and nervous system to include autoimmune phenomena of every kind. As always, the major obstacle remains the dearth of reliable statistics, the systematic underreporting of adverse vaccine events, and the overly rigid criteria for inclusion in the CDC figures, based on the standards and guidelines set by the industry.

Chapter 6

BRAIN DAMAGE

Encompassing the entire spectrum of neurological impairment in children, the authentic "smoking gun" of autoimmune brain and central nervous system damage attributable to vaccines includes encephalopathy, encephalitis, Guillain-Barré syndrome, seizures, learning disabilities, sensory processing disorder, mental retardation, ADD and ADHD, and autism. To get some idea of the magnitude of the problem, here are the official CDC figures for the most prevalent of these, making due allowance for the fact that by no means all of the cases are vaccine-related, and the proportion of those that are remains unknown and indeed hotly contested:[1]

Learning and developmental disabilities	1 in 6	16.7%
ADD and ADHD	1 in 10	10.0%
Autism	1 in 45	2.2%
TOTAL		**28.9%**

Notwithstanding that uncertainty, it remains a shocking statistic that more than a quarter of all American children and adolescents alive today suffer from some form of brain injury or illness. Since almost every child is multiply vaccinated, and it is known for certain that every vaccine *can* produce brain damage in susceptible individuals, the obvious question for science is to determine how many of these cases are vaccine-related and autoimmune in nature.

DPT ENCEPHALOPATHY

Although the exact tally is not known, an unprecedented number of personal injury lawsuits, certainly many hundreds and probably thousands, were brought against vaccine manufacturers throughout the 1980s on behalf of children who had died or suffered severe, permanent brain damage shortly after being vaccinated; in a significant minority of these cases, the courts ruled in their favor and compensated them generously for their injuries.

During those years, most attention was focused on the DPT and DTP vaccines, and the whole-cell pertussis component in particular; the diverse neuropathologies attributed to it were lumped together into the wastebasket category "DPT encephalopathy," encompassing all types and degrees of mental and developmental retardation and impairment, including seizures, learning disabilities, and autism.

Here is a representative case from that era, that of a three-year-old girl whose mother wrote to me requesting an affidavit in support of her litigation against the child's doctors and the Canadian government:

> Our beautiful daughter was damaged as a result of her 18-month vaccination, which consisted of the DPT, Hib, and oral polio vaccines. One week later, she had a bizarre screaming episode, and is now labeled "autistic," or PDD. Last month we took her to the Mayo Clinic, where an MRI showed brain inflammation and demyelination. One of the doctors admitted to us privately that she suffers from post-vaccine encephalitis.
>
> She had maybe 25 words at 18 months, and was ahead in some developmental milestones, as well as being quite social. Immediately after her screaming episode, she stopped talking, and began ignoring the neighborhood kids and making no eye contact. As new parents, we first thought her behavior was "just a phase," but then she developed hand-flapping and other repetitive, stereotyped behaviors as well.
>
> We realized we had a serious problem, and told her pediatrician that we suspected her 18-month vaccinations were the cause. He agreed that she was autistic, and sent her to specialists for further evaluation. We insisted that she had changed abruptly after the vaccinations, and showed them a video of her as an infant and toddler in which she seemed perfectly normal; and they agreed. From photos taken before and after, the damage is obvious: her eyes have lost their gleam, and she looks sad and alone. We were very persistent, but her doctors dismissed it as a coincidence, and no further mention of any vaccine was ever included in their reports.[2]

Apart from the extremity of this girl's misfortune, what impressed me most was both her pediatrician's and various specialists' unanimous dismissal of even the possibility that it could have been caused by the vaccinations, exemplifying a shared, quasi-religious faith that I've already commented on, and has never ceased to amaze me.

I wrote a letter on the girl's behalf, because I felt sure that the abrupt and dramatic change documented in her photos and video would carry enough weight with a jury to overrule the standard defense argument that the shattered promise of this girl's life was simply an unfortunate coincidence for which nobody was responsible. I never learned the outcome.

Another case from the same era was that of a three-year-old boy who had reacted badly to his first DPT and eventually began to recover, but then suffered grievous and permanent brain damage after the second. Once again, I learned of it in a letter, this time from the lawyer who represented him in his parents' suit against the manufacturer, likewise requesting an affidavit:

> Our firm represents a child who was born normal and healthy in every way. After his first DPT at six weeks, he began falling off growth charts, exhibited multiple developmental delays, and was diagnosed as "failure to thrive," but then slowly began to recover. At five months he received his second DPT, and his delays became much more extreme. He has never recovered.
>
> He is now three years old, with the mental capacity of an infant of a year and a half. I am convinced that his problems came about as a result of the DPT. In view of what happened after the first shot, he should not have had the second, or at least the pertussis component of it.[3]

Here, too, I was happy to write the letter without a face-to-face meeting, because its tragic pattern of a warning ignored, a lesser version with eventual recovery, followed by death or irreversible brain damage after a repeat dose, tallied so closely with my own clinical experience. It was also a prominent feature of the exposé *DPT: a Shot in the Dark,* in which the medical historian Harris Coulter and Barbara Loe Fisher, whose infant son had been damaged by the vaccine, painstakingly collected the stories of more than one hundred little victims.[4]

The public outcry over these DPT cases impelled Ms. Fisher and a friend with her own brain-injured child to found Dissatisfied Parents Together, or DPT, which rapidly grew to become the National Vaccine Information Center (NVIC), a support and advocacy group for families and friends of vaccine-injured children that still hosts conferences, publishes a newsletter and educational materials, and maintains a large database and an extensive network of local chapters all over the country. After testifying before Congress, Ms. Fisher also helped write the National Childhood Vaccine Injury Act of 1986, which created the VAERS reporting system and the VICP program for compensating injury claims as an alternative to litigation.

A large part of the controversy regarding DPT encephalopathy focuses on the statistics for its prevalence, which are notoriously inexact, in part because of the vagueness of its definition, its overly restrictive link to the DPT, and the tendency to ignore conditions taking longer to develop, as we saw. A final source of uncertainty arises from the large and essentially unstudied population of damaged children whose parents never report the injury and never sue for damages, yet another source of invisibility that dovetails with all the other factors and adds another large unknown to the total.

The First DPT Encephalopathy Study

These difficulties were already evident in the classic study conducted by Professor Gordon Stewart of Glasgow University, who tried to establish the exact incidence of brain damage from the pertussis vaccine in that area of Scotland before 1979, mainly to test the prevailing assumption that the risk of death or severe damage from the vaccine was far outweighed by that from the disease itself. What he found was quite the opposite,

1. that adverse reactions were more common and more serious than had generally been recognized;
2. that current schedules of vaccination were ineffective in preventing the disease; and
3. that epidemiological monitoring of efficacy and adverse reactions was incomplete.[5]

Out of a total of 270,000 children vaccinated between 1968 and 1972, he found only 5 recorded cases of brain damage after the DPT, for an incidence of 1 in 54,000 children; but after persistent inquiries he uncovered a sizable number of additional deaths and brain injuries that were not reported, from which he surmised that there were still more of whom he had no knowledge.[6] In the process, he also learned that the incidence and severity of the natural disease, which had been declining rapidly in the decades before vaccination, continued to do so at roughly the same pace, so that the vaccine could not be shown to be effective in any bottom-line sense.[7]

Finally, he painstakingly delineated the signs and symptoms of the "pertussis reaction syndrome," as he called it, which dovetailed perfectly with the cases of DPT encephalopathy described so movingly in Coulter and Fisher's book.[8] Most of all, his reliance on the clinical perspective, with its insistence on paying attention to the actual experience of real individuals, conveys the enormity of their loss, regardless of the statistics. His final words on the subject seem especially germane and even prescient today:

> Because of the national deficit in epidemiological data, it is impossible to estimate the prevalence of subsequent brain damage and mental defect. It is unlikely to be lower than 1 in 60,000, but might be 1 in 10,000, or even higher. If it is 1 in 20,000, say, then 30 children will suffer permanent brain damage in the UK each year, and many more might be started on the early stages of an organic dementia which in its final form has the features of a demyelinating disease. This risk far exceeds the present risk of death or permanent damage from whooping-cough, or even, in some parts of the country, from the chance of contracting it.[9]

A Moral Question

Implicitly, he is asking the same moral question that we should all be asking, whether we are prepared to tolerate even a small number of dead and brain-damaged children, while knowing in advance that the vaccine will cause them, that the risk is greater than that of the natural disease, that the deaths and injuries are wholly preventable by simply not vaccinating, and that the choice would be somewhat less onerous if the vaccine were not required, but simply made available to those who still want it after being fully informed of the risks.

Given that the United States is a much more populous country, we may suppose that mandating the DTP or DTaP means accepting 100 cases a year, or 1,000, or 10,000, as the case may be, in the same casual manner that we condone the "collateral damage" of innocent men, women, and children killed in a drone strike against easily misidentified shapes on a faraway screen that we hire technicians to treat as our enemies. Oddly enough, our ongoing commitment to the DTaP implies that sacrificing a small number of our children's lives every year for the greater good is negligible; yet the mere possibility of *saving* 100 lives annually was deemed sufficient justification for vaccinating the entire population against chicken pox and rotavirus against their will.[10] Instead, I would argue, both atrocities raise a basic moral issue that far outweighs any such calculus.

Understated CDC Estimates

Regarding the DTP and DTaP alone, the VICP website provides the following statistics for serious adverse reactions between October 1988 and June 2015:

- For the DTP, 3286 claims of injury and 696 of death, for a total of 3982 claims, of which 1271 were compensated and 2706 were dismissed;
- For the DTaP, 382 claims of injury and 79 of death, for a total of 461 claims, of which 185 were compensated and 205 were dismissed.[11]

Although these figures also include other reactions, notably anaphylaxis, encephalopathy heads the list in the frequency of complications severe enough to prompt legal action. If we accept the educated guess of Dr. David Kessler, former head of the FDA, that only about 1% of them are ever reported,[12] simply multiplying these figures by 100 would yield a figure of roughly 330,000 injuries after the DTP of sufficient severity to warrant a VICP claim, plus about 70,000 deaths, as well as about 40,000 injuries from the DTaP and 8000 deaths.

These numbers also appear to suggest that the newer, acellular DTaP has lowered the incidence of death and severe adverse reactions to the vaccine significantly, as it was intended to do. But since the FDA and CDC admit that only 1%, or at most 10%, of the serious reactions are actually reported, and the vast majority of VICP claims for damages based on them are dismissed, it is not difficult to understand why fewer and fewer aggrieved parents even bother to file a claim. Nor can anybody plausibly argue that these difficulties are unintentional, since we do know very precisely whom we've vaccinated and how many doses we've given them, so that recording their injuries and compensating them decently for the misery we have caused them would require little more than simply paying closer attention to the infrastructure that is already in place.

The Campaign to Discredit DPT Encephalopathy

Even though if not precisely because it was the basis for most of the court settlements and a driving force behind the VICP program, the entity of "DPT encephalopathy" was repeatedly and vociferously attacked throughout the 1990s by some of the most influential physicians of the pro-vaccine lobby.

In 1990, for example, Dr. Edward Mortimer, et al., published a review in the *Journal of the AMA* that claimed, "No child who was previously normal without a prior history had a seizure in the 3 days following a DPT vaccine that marked the onset of epilepsy or other neurological or developmental abnormality. Our negative findings reinforce those of previous investigators that serious neurological events are rarely if ever caused by DPT."[13]

In the lead editorial of the same issue, Dr. James Cherry, another leading vaccine advocate whom we've met before, cited these data as conclusive proof that "DPT encephalopathy" is essentially a myth, based on a "coincidence," and should therefore be erased once and for all from the ever-shrinking list of genuine adverse reactions meriting compensation:

> In recent months, three controlled studies examined the risk of seizures and other acute neurological illnesses after DPT, involving 230,000 children and 713,000 vaccinations. These studies found no evidence of a causal link between the DPT and permanent neurological illness. It is not surprising that physicians tended to blame the vaccine for these events. But these recent studies show that the major problem has been failure to separate sequences from consequences. It is late in the 20th century, and it's time for the myth of "DPT encephalopathy" to end.[14]

Somewhat more judiciously, the same objection was raised by a 1996 report of the CDC's Advisory Committee on Immunization Practices, likewise dominated by physicians promoting mandatory vaccination, which professed sympathy for the plight of devastated parents, but then cast doubt on the legitimacy of their claims by bogging them down in a veritable swamp of evasions, equivocations, and official bureaucratese:

> Rare but serious acute neurological illnesses, including encephalitis, encephalopathy, and convulsions, have been reported following DPT. The National Child Encephalopathy Study provides evidence that DPT can cause encephalopathy. This occurs rarely, but detailed follow-up indicates that children who developed a serious neurological illness after DPT were significantly more likely than children in the control group to have chronic CNS dysfunction ten years later and to have been given DPT within seven days of its onset.
>
> The ACIP proposed 3 possible explanations for this association:
>
> 1. The dysfunction could have been caused by DPT.
> 2. DPT could trigger events in children with brain or metabolic abnormalities who might also experience them if other stimuli such as fever or infection are present.
> 3. DPT might cause the event in children with underlying abnormalities who would have become dysfunctional even without it.

> The data do not support any one explanation over the others. The evidence was consistent with a causal relationship, but insufficient to determine whether DPT increases the overall risk ten years later.[15]

These hair-splitting distinctions seemed to accept a causal link only in the absence of any underlying predisposition, in spite of the self-evident truth that *all* illnesses presuppose both external morbid stimuli and individuals capable of receiving and responding to them in their own way. This is precisely the great, overarching riddle of clinical medicine, which the benighted quest for totally effective and necessary causes without preexisting tendencies either quietly glosses over or unscrupulously hides behind, as the occasion demands.

In practice, the distinction is useless and inconsistent, since patients showing a strong family history of adverse reactions to vaccines, for example, are obviously in a much higher risk pool than others, yet are often *not* exempted, while genuinely rare, life-threatening emergencies, like anaphylaxis, representing the highest possible extreme of individual susceptibility, have been accepted onto the list without question, the main difference between them being simply that the former predisposition was known in advance, while the latter was not.

Equally artificial is the ACIP's distinction between reactions "caused" by the vaccine and those merely "triggered" by it, since every reaction presupposes some degree of receptivity, whether known in advance or not, and our patients may lie almost anywhere on this continuum, depending on genetics, epigenetics, and circumstances alike. The third possibility, an underlying predisposition that would have manifested later even without the vaccine, is meaningless in logic as well as science, since the vaccine-related event is a *fait accompli* that has already occurred and thus preempts any possible real-world test of its validity.

In any case, no matter which of the three official explanations is chosen, the bottom line remains the same: a patient has been vaccinated and suffered a major injury or developed a significant chronic illness not long afterward, which the victim, parent, physician, or guardian rightly or wrongly attributes to the vaccination. That is the riddle that must be solved in each case; and once again the irony is that the clinical perspective, that is, simply paying attention to the individual patient, as physicians are trained to do, offers a far more reliable means of solving it than any statistical guideline, or the tidy little list of complications so far identified, or the ACIP's three distinctions, none of which properly qualifies as a mere coincidence.

In spite of this prolonged and determined opposition, encephalopathy remains on the official government list of reportable and compensable adverse reactions from the acellular DTaP vaccine, which does seem to have lowered the official risk of brain damage at least to the extent that the pro-vaccine lobby has finally made its peace with it; so it is now duly listed as an adverse reaction in the package insert.

In any case, while awards for DPT encephalopathy have declined over the past twenty years, the same interval has seen a dramatic increase in the number of mandated vaccines, a newfound awareness that some form of brain damage can result from any one or combination of them, and a growing body of evidence that the mercury preservative thimerosal, adjuvants like aluminum, and the autoimmune mechanisms they are known to cause are certainly responsible for many cases. But even as late as 2011, the DTP and DTaP still accounted for more than half of the $2 billion so far awarded to victims under the VICP program.

MMR AND AUTISM

In 1943, the psychiatrist Leo Kanner, MD, described in detail a number of children exhibiting a previously unrecognized ensemble of signs and symptoms, including bizarre gestures and mannerisms, aversion to company and asocial behavior, and sometimes astonishing feats of memory, to which he gave the name "autism."[16] At first, the syndrome was included under the broad umbrella of "encephalopathy," or brain damage, but remained relatively uncommon as a separate diagnosis in its own right until the mid- and late 1990s, when many new vaccines were mandated, new cases were identified on an unprecedented scale, and "autism" began to be talked about more widely in public health circles.

The Wakefield Saga

The first breakthrough came in 1995, when Andrew Wakefield, MD, a British gastroenterologist studying autoimmune inflammatory bowel disease, published a retrospective study in the *Lancet,* comparing 3,550 adults who had received the measles vaccine as infants with 11,400 of their peers who had not.[17] To his amazement, the vaccinated group was found to be three times more likely than their unvaccinated controls to develop Crohn's disease later in life, and twice as likely to develop ulcerative colitis.[18] Strangely enough, this shocking finding received comparatively little attention on either side of the pond; and as far as I'm aware, nobody has ever refuted or even challenged it.

But its effect on Dr. Wakefield himself was life-changing. In 1998, he published a series of follow-up experiments with several colleagues that created a worldwide sensation, prompted the *Lancet* to retract the article based on their findings, caused the lead investigators to lose their jobs and medical licenses, and has already changed medical history.

Eight children with a history of normal development who developed autism or encephalitis soon after their MMR vaccination were referred to Dr. Wakefield's clinic for GI evaluation because of additional signs and symptoms of enterocolitis. Biopsies of the ileum and colon revealed lymphoid hyperplasia in a pattern characteristic of Crohn's disease and ulcerative colitis, both major autoimmune diseases; but, as he was very careful to say,

> We did not prove an association between MMR vaccine and the syndrome described. Virological studies are underway that may help to resolve this issue. If there is a causal link between the vaccine and the syndrome, a rising incidence might be anticipated after the introduction of this vaccine to the UK in 1988. Published evidence is inadequate to show whether this is a change in incidence or a link to the vaccine.[19]

Two years later, he gave sworn testimony to a committee of the US Congress that the virological studies he had spoken of had indeed revealed antibodies to measles in these lymphocyte aggregations, but not to mumps, rubella, or other viruses, and that such patients were subsequently found to be less able than age-matched, unvaccinated controls to respond normally to other common antigens to which they had previously been exposed, such as the DPT vaccine, dust mites, and *Candida albicans*, and more prone to asthma, hay fever, eczema, otitis media, and URIs as well.[20] Still, he made no claim that MMR was "the cause" of autism, and indeed went no further than recommending that its measles, mumps, and rubella components be administered separately.

The Campaign to Discredit Him

Notwithstanding the restraint of his language and the moderation of his claims, the evidence he presented made him a marked man for the vaccine industry and their physician-advocates in both Britain and the United States. Almost immediately, a new crop of epidemiological studies were published that loudly and unanimously denied any causal link between the MMR vaccine and autism.[21] In 2001, he relocated to the United States, after having been removed from his position at the London hospital where his research had been conducted.

Beginning in 2003, the *British Medical Journal* commissioned Brian Deer, a reporter for the *Sunday Times* of London, to investigate every aspect of Wakefield's life and career. Deer's ongoing, award-winning defamations were serialized in the *BMJ*, and republished in a number of news outlets in the United States and United Kingdom.[22] Some of the most serious accusations were that Wakefield had limited his studies to patients handpicked by the lawyer representing them in a pending damage lawsuit against the vaccine manufacturers, and had been paid handsomely in secret for doing so; that he falsified his data; and that his research had never been replicated elsewhere.[23]

Meanwhile, no doubt prompted at least in part by Deer's work, the *Lancet* mounted its own investigations to determine if its ethical standards had been violated. Although the sources of their complaints were not specified, they dutifully mined the terrain that Deer had already mapped out, namely,

1. that prior ethical approval was not obtained for invasive procedures performed on some of the children, contrary to what the article claimed;
2. that prior ethical approval was obtained for a study that was entirely different from the one that the article was based on;
3. that the children studied were not consecutively referred to the GI clinic, as the article claimed, but invited by the authors to participate in it, based on their parents' belief in a causal link to the vaccine;
4. that the children were part of a group project funded by Legal Aid to seek grounds for pursuing legal action against the vaccine manufacturer on their behalf, a project headed by Dr. Wakefield and not disclosed to the journal;
5. that the results of the study were in fact used in subsequent legal action, begun prior to publication, and likewise not disclosed to the journal; and
6. that Dr. Wakefield was paid £55,000 by the Legal Aid Board for his work, including the study, which thus represented a conflict of financial interest that should have been disclosed but was not.[24]

To his credit, Dr. Richard Horton, the editor in chief, ruled that the first three allegations were without merit;[25] but he upheld the remaining allegations that there was indeed a conflict of interest that should have been reported, and that might well have influenced him not to publish the article if it had been:

> Dr. Wakefield had two roles. He was the lead investigator in the study of a new syndrome of bowel and psychiatric symptoms. He was also commissioned by a lawyer to undertake virological investigations as part of a study funded by Legal Aid. When he submitted his 1998 paper, this second study was not disclosed, and should have been, even though many of the children were involved in both studies, which also involved different aspects of his work. Because of that dual role, the perception of a conflict of interest remains.[26]

His Victory

To make a long story short, Wakefield's 1998 article was formally retracted, for one of the very few times in the journal's more than century-long history. Although the verdict seems unnecessarily harsh, Dr. Wakefield must have known that his Legal Aid work would be perceived as a conflict of interest, and suspected that Horton might reject the article if this hidden agenda were revealed, as Horton's own statement later confirmed.

In other words, rather than being simply the innocent victim of a witch hunt, the default assumption among his supporters, perhaps he deliberately chose to run that risk, in spite of knowing that he might well be disciplined for it, because it was the only possible way for his all-important findings to be made public under the circumstances. The result was a witch hunt just the same; but I admire him all the more for doing what was right and necessary and suffering the consequences, gratuitously cruel though they were. From that vantage point, what he did and how he did it achieved a tremendous victory for mankind, both for science and for speaking the truth, however rarely acknowledged as such.

In 2010, the UK General Medical Council's own disciplinary investigation concluded by revoking Dr. Wakefield's license to practice, along with that of his senior colleague, Dr. John Walker-Smith.[27] To disprove Deer's accusation that he and Wakefield had fabricated their evidence, Walker-Smith revealed that he himself had presented findings of autism and autoimmune enterocolitis in the children who participated in the study well before Wakefield's involvement in it, and was therefore duly exonerated.[28]

As for Wakefield, the American medical community has still not forgiven him for the mere suggestion that the triple MMR might have been responsible in some cases; but he has since become a featured speaker at conferences in the United States and abroad, an outspoken advocate for the cause of safer vaccines and parental choice, and the beloved hero and worthy champion of the parents of vaccine-injured children everywhere who look to him for inspiration, guidance, and comfort in their bottomless pit of grief and travail.

Meanwhile, relying on the same research expressly undertaken to refute his findings, the medical establishment in both countries has continued to deny any causal link between the MMR and autism, and to congratulate itself that Wakefield's perceived threat to their reigning mythology has been disposed of, seemingly ignorant of the fact that his biopsy findings have been repeatedly confirmed by other investigators,[29] as has his observation that the UK, which uses the same diagnostic criteria that we do, reported a dramatic and almost identical increase in the rate of autism cases ten years after our own, beginning at precisely the time when the MMR vaccine was introduced on a mass scale in Britain.[30]

It bears repeating that his article was retracted and his license revoked solely on the basis of the alleged conflict of interest, not because of his biopsy specimens and virological findings, the objective validity of which remains intact and unchallenged, no matter how his subjects were selected. Moreover, largely in response to his work, the same combination of autistic and other forms of brain damage, enterocolitis, and food and environmental allergies has been reported by large numbers of parents throughout the United States, the UK, Canada, Australia, Western Europe, and parts of Asia,[31] while integrative physicians in the United States have published many case reports to show that relieving the allergies and GI symptoms with natural methods such as vitamins, supplements, and diet have proved beneficial for the autistic syndromes as well.[32]

But the ultimate refutation of these smug denials has recently come from deep inside the heart of the medical establishment itself, from revelations by a CDC scientist that the agency knew for at least 15 years that the MMR posed a significant risk of autism and deliberately buried the information, as we shall see, while even the dreaded Vaccine Court, heavily weighted against victims though it remains, has begun to make awards in a few particularly egregious cases.[33]

THE FAST-GROWING EPIDEMIC OF BRAIN DAMAGE

Meanwhile, as even the CDC has admitted, the incidence of autism in the United States has continued to rise continuously and indeed precipitously since the 1980s, as shown in the table below.

1 in 2000,	or 0.05%,	in 1983,	to
1 in 150,	or 0.67%,	in 2000,	to
1 in 110,	or 0.91%,	in 2006,	to
1 in 88,	or 1.13%,	in 2008,	to
1 in 68,	or 1.47%,	in 2010,	to
1 in 45,	or 2.22%,	in 2014.[34]	

This represents a roughly 40-fold increase, which the agency has never explained or even appeared to take much interest in, dismissing it as an artifact of the generally heightened awareness of and more exact criteria for the autism spectrum in the medical community, the schools, and the public, resulting in more frequent and accurate diagnosis.

But even if that explanation were true, the agency has remained studiedly mute about the phenomenon itself—the scandalous fact that a shocking and rapidly growing proportion of all children born in the United States, at present more than 2%, suffer from a major autoimmune, neurodevelopmental disability that has required and will continue to require intensive medical, psychological, and educational therapy and other assistance throughout their lives, at enormous expense to their parents and the taxpayers alike.

At the very least, this elephant in the room represents a public health crisis of enormous proportions that cries out for precisely the sort of comprehensive and intelligent inquiry that physicians and public health officials seem reluctant if not positively unwilling to undertake, in view of which their blanket official assurances have become increasingly hollow and difficult even for their own sworn followers to accept.

Such at least was the opinion of Bernardine Healy, MD, the highly respected former head of the National Institutes of Health, who raised something of a furor in a 2009 interview merely by admitting that a causal link with vaccines is *possible,* and therefore deserves more serious investigation than it has yet received:

> I think that public health officials have been too quick to dismiss the hypothesis as irrational. They don't want to pursue a hypothesis that could be damaging to public health by scaring people. I don't think you should turn your back on a scientific hypothesis because you're afraid of what it might reveal. What we're seeing is that in the bulk of the population vaccines are safe, but there may be this susceptible group. The fact that you don't want to know them is

> a real disappointment to me. If you turn your back on that possibility, what can I say?[35]

Moreover, the total incidence of neurodevelopmental injury and disability in children is, in fact, a whole order of magnitude higher than the CDC's estimate, since the abstract diagnosis "Autism Spectrum Disorder," or ASD, is merely an important subset of the epidemic of brain damage, involving a broad spectrum of diagnoses and clinical presentations that pediatricians and family physicians encounter on a daily basis. The DSM-V, the current *Diagnostic and Statistical Manual of Mental Disorders,* lists the following diagnostic criteria for ASD:

1. Deficits in social communication, interaction, reciprocity, interests, emotions, affect, and responses;
2. Deficits in nonverbal communication, eye contact, body language, gestures, facial expression, or understanding;
3. Deficits in relationships, sharing play, making friends, or interest in peers;
4. Stereotyped or repetitive movements, such as echolalia, repeated phrases, lining up toys, insistence on sameness, inflexible adherence to routines or ritualized behavior;
5. Highly restricted, fixated interests of abnormal focus and intensity; and
6. Hyper- or hyporeactivity to sensory input (sounds, textures, smells, light).[36]

Sometimes overlapping with ASD but characterized somewhat differently and diagnosed separately in most cases, other neurodevelopmental problems commonly seen in children include ADD and ADHD, which are almost five times more prevalent than ASD; "Intellectual Developmental Disorder" and "Global Developmental Delay," roughly corresponding to "encephalopathy" and "mental and developmental retardation," as brain damage from the DPT was formerly described; "Communication Disorders," involving deficits in speech, language, and/or social communication; "Specific Learning Disorder," involving reading, writing, reasoning, etc., formerly lumped together as "learning disabilities"; "Sensory Processing Disorder"; and finally, "Motor Disorders," including deficits in coordination, stereotypic movements, tics, and Tourette's syndrome.[37]

If vaccines are indeed causally linked to autism and ASD, as a growing body of scientific research clearly indicates, purely on logical grounds it is reasonable to suspect that they will sooner or later be linked to these other forms of brain damage as well, a conclusion that my own clinical impression and I daresay the experience of most pediatricians would tend to support as well. If so, the incidence figures will have to be raised by at least a whole order of magnitude to include the entire vast spectrum of neurodevelopmental and neuropsychiatric disabilities in children.

THIMEROSAL AND ALUMINUM

In any case, it is eloquent testimony to the CDC's real agenda that, even in 2015, its home page on Vaccine Safety still dutifully adhered to the official line, in spite of everything that has come to light in the past fifteen years, not least from scandals within the Agency itself:

> Autism spectrum disorder (ASD) is a developmental disability that is caused by differences in how the brain functions. Recent estimates have found that about 1 in 68 children have been identified with ASD in communities across the United States. *Studies have shown that there is no link between vaccines and autism.*
>
> *Vaccine ingredients do not cause autism.* One ingredient that has been studied is Thimerosal, a mercury-based preservative used to prevent contamination. A 2004 scientific review by the Institute of Medicine concluded that "the evidence favors rejection of a causal relationship between Thimerosal–containing vaccines and autism." Since 2003, nine CDC-funded studies have found no link between Thimerosal-containing vaccines or the MMR vaccine and ASD in children.[38]

The CDC has never wavered from this claim, in splendid contempt for all the science that has questioned or doubted it for the past fifteen years at least, much of it implicating thimerosal in particular. Partly as a result of these studies, the public outcry that followed, and a number of Congressional hearings on the subject, thimerosal was quietly removed from or reduced to trace amounts in all vaccines except for influenza; but the CDC has never recognized these studies, and would have us believe that the mercury was taken out purely as a precaution:

> Between 1999 and 2001, Thimerosal was removed or reduced to trace amounts in all childhood vaccines except for some flu vaccines. This was done as part of a broader national effort to reduce mercury exposure in children as a precaution, before studies determined that Thimerosal was not harmful.[39]

Edited by Robert F. Kennedy Jr., the nephew of JFK, the 2014 book *Thimerosal: Let the Science Speak* ably recounts this history in abundant detail.[40]

The following is a brief summary of some scientific studies that have supported a causal linkage between autism and thimerosal and may have played a role in its removal:

1. A 2009 study of male newborns receiving hepatitis B vaccine containing thimerosal within the first month of life, which demonstrated roughly triple the incidence of autism when compared to that of unvaccinated controls;[41]
2. A 2006 study that showed that even minute amounts of thimerosal interfere with cytokine signaling in neurons, thus causing immune dysregulation;[42]
3. A 2005 study that documented accumulation of thimerosal in the brain at twice the levels of methylmercury, itself a well-known neurotoxin;[43]
4. A 2004 study showing inhibited methylation by mercury and aluminum as a possible mechanism for their neurodevelopmental toxicity;[44]
5. A 2007 study that correlated the intensity of autistic signs and symptoms with concentrations of mercury in blood and hair;[45]
6. A 2007 study of nine autistic children, of whom eight were found to have developed ASD after receiving thimerosal-containing vaccines, to have excreted excessive amounts of mercury following chelation, and the severity of whose ASD picture was proportional to the total dose of mercury they received;[46] and
7. A 2006 study from Hong Kong that demonstrated high levels of mercury in the blood of children with ADHD when compared with matched normal children.[47]

As we saw, mercury is by no means the whole story, since autism has also developed in children who received no thimerosal in their vaccines, notably the MMR, which has remained a prime suspect in autism ever since Dr. Wakefield's work. The following are summaries of various studies providing evidence linking autism to other vaccines, to the vaccination process in general, and to exposure to environmental toxins generally:

8. A 2006 French study that demonstrated high levels of coproporphyrin in the urine of autistic children as compared with normal controls, indicating that autism represents some form of environmental toxicity;[48]

9. A 2011 review of autistic cases from 1943 on that were linked to genetic mutations or deletions or some form of environmental toxic exposure, the latter exemplified mainly by encephalitis with viral infections or after vaccination;[49]
10. A 2005 study of cases that showed ASD to be much broader than simply a neuropsychiatric disturbance, also encompassing a global immune dysregulation, inflammatory bowel disease, and increased susceptibility to infections and inflammations generally;[50]
11. A 2005 study of cases validating the original autistic regression through comparing home videos taken at 12 and 24 months of age;[51]
12. A 2006 study of autistic children at a special-needs center that detected a chemical marker of impaired oxidative phosphorylation, a sign of mitochondrial dysfunction, in 38% of the subjects, and another different marker of the same deficiency in another 47%, which pointed to "oxidative stress" as a basic mechanism of the brain damage seen in autism;[52]
13. A 2007 study that showed the aluminum adjuvant used in many vaccines to be highly toxic to motor neurons in the brain and spinal cord;[53]
14. A 2003 study of autism in California that refuted the argument of its dramatic increase being an artifact of improved diagnosis;[54] and
15. A 2008 study that showed autism to be essentially a mitochondrial disease, resulting from exposure to environmental toxins, and causing oxidative stress.[55]

In short, there is a great deal of published scientific work indicating that the brain damage seen in autism

1. is only an important part of a global autoimmune dysfunction that also affects many other tissues and organ systems, especially the GI tract, precisely as Dr. Wakefield first pointed out long ago;
2. is characterized by oxidative stress, mitochondrial dysfunction, and autoimmune dysregulation and inflammation throughout the body; and
3. is brought about by exposure to environmental toxins, including and especially vaccines, but by no means exclusively limited to them.

THE CDC COVER-UP

If all that scientific evidence is still insufficient to convince some people, the last few years have added incontrovertible proof of deception at the highest levels of the vaccine establishment, as many have long suspected, namely, to the effect that the CDC and the vaccine manufacturers have known for decades that vaccines cause autism, but conspired to hide the evidence, and that the studies they habitually cite to deny such a link were fraudulent, having been commissioned for the sole purpose of misleading the public.

In 2014, William Thompson, PhD, a senior research scientist at the CDC, issued a press release in which he admitted that a 2004 study claiming that the MMR vaccine did not cause autism had suppressed data showing quite the opposite, namely, a 340% increase in autism among black males who received the MMR before the age of 36 months:

> I regret that my coauthors and I omitted statistically significant information in our 2004 article published in the journal *Pediatrics.* The omitted data suggested that African-American males who received the MMR vaccine before age 36 months were at increased risk for autism. Decisions were made regarding which findings to report after the data were collected. I believe it is the responsibility of the CDC to properly convey the risks associated with the receipt of those vaccines.[56]

In subsequent written testimony that he provided to Rep. William Posey (R-Florida), Dr. Thompson confessed that he and his coworkers were ordered to destroy the data from the study by their two superiors at the agency, both senior executives at the CDC's Safety Division:

> The study co-authors scheduled a meeting to destroy documents related to the study, brought a big garbage can into the meeting room, went through and reviewed all the hard-copy documents that we thought we should discard, and put them into the can. Because I assumed it was illegal and would violate both the Freedom of Information Act and Department of Justice requests, I kept hard copy of all documents in my office, and I retain all associated computer files.
>
> I have great shame now when I meet a family with kids with autism, because I've been part of the problem. Because the CDC has not been transparent, we've missed ten years of research. They're not doing what they should be doing; they're afraid to look for things that might be associated. The higher-ups wanted to do certain things and I went along with it.[57]

Granted Congressional immunity for his testimony, Dr. Thompson made it clear beyond any reasonable doubt that the CDC not only knew about the substantial risk of autism posed by the MMR for at least fifteen years, and emphatically denied that there was any risk at all, but thereby also knowingly condemned a large but still carefully hidden number of American children to become autistic as a result, as well as putting millions more unknowingly at risk.

Even before Dr. Thompson's sensational revelations, anonymous leaks from within the Agency revealed that the CDC had also commissioned and funded a study of Danish schoolchildren that falsely claimed the incidence of autism rose significantly after Denmark *removed* thimerosal from its vaccines,[58] even though the authors were well aware that the real reason was the new policy of the Danish government to list all autism cases on a National Registry for the first time.[59] Compiled by senior CDC officials and their Vaccine Safety Datalink Team, several versions of this intentionally misleading data were published in prestigious medical journals in the United States, including one in *Pediatrics* that was endlessly cited by the agency to assure the medical community and the news media that thimerosal was safe and did not cause autism,[60] a finding that was greeted with almost unanimous relief and uncritically passed off as scientific fact by the medical community as a whole.

But investigative reporters like Robert F. Kennedy Jr. and Sharyl Attkisson of *CBS News* learned that Dr. Poul Thorsen, one of the lead authors of the original Danish study, had been hired by the CDC for the sole purpose of demolishing the link between vaccines and autism, and had conducted several other studies of the same type, for which the Agency continued to pay him handsomely until he went missing in 2010, after being indicted in Denmark and the United States for having embezzled several million dollars from Aarhus University:

> Danish police are investigating Dr. Poul Thorsen, who has vanished along with almost $2 million that he had supposedly spent on research. Thorsen was a leading member of a Danish research group that wrote several key studies supporting CDC claims that the MMR vaccine and mercury-laden vaccines were safe for children. His 2003 study reported a 20-fold increase in autism after Denmark *banned* mercury preservative in its vaccines, and concluded that mercury could not be behind the autism epidemic.
>
> His study has been criticized as fraudulent since it failed to disclose that the increase was an artifact of new mandates requiring that autism cases be reported on the national registry. Despite this obvious chicanery, CDC has long touted the study as the proof that mercury-laced vaccines are safe for infants

> and young children. Mainstream media have also relied on it as the basis for its public assurances that it is safe to inject young children with mercury at concentrations hundreds of times over U.S. safety limits.
>
> Thorsen parlayed that study into a long-term relationship with CDC, and built a research empire that advertised its close association with the CDC autism team, while the agency paid Thorsen and his staff millions of dollars to churn out research papers, many reassuring the public on vaccine safety. The discovery of his fraud came from an investigation by Aarhus University and the CDC, which discovered that he had falsified documents and accepted salaries in violation of university rules from the Danish university, and from Emory University in Atlanta, near CDC headquarters. Thorsen's center has received $14.6 million from CDC since 2002.
>
> His partner Kreesten Madsen recently came under fierce criticism after damning e-mails surfaced showing Madsen and CDC officials fraudulently cherry-picking facts to prove vaccine safety. Leading independent scientists have accused CDC of concealing the link between the dramatic increases in mercury-laced child vaccinations beginning in 1989 and the epidemic of autism, neurological disorders, and other illnesses affecting every generation of American children since. Questions about Thorsen's scientific integrity may finally force CDC to rethink its vaccine protocols, since most pro-vaccine studies cited by CDC rely on the findings of his research group, published in the *Journal of the AMA*, the *American Journal of Preventive Medicine*, the American Academy of Pediatrics, the *New England Journal of Medicine* and others. The validity of all these studies is now in question.[61]

As well as documenting the occurrence of these deceptions and cover-ups, and the ruined lives that they caused, these revelations are no less profoundly shocking for the muted, circumspect, and indeed virtually nonexistent reaction they have elicited from the medical profession and the general public, allowing the CDC to continue adhering to its official line, the mainstream media to continue censoring themselves without having to be told, and most parents to continue vaccinating their children as if nothing had happened. As with the Iraqi invasion and the financial collapse, it is as though we have become so inured to official lies and corruption at the highest level that those who insist on vaccination while knowing the risks and keeping them secret have not only escaped punishment, but continue to enjoy the same level of prestige and esteem as before.

SUMMARY

Approximately one-quarter of all children in the United States now suffer from encephalopathy, autism, ADD, ADHD, a learning disability, or some form of brain damage, which the best contemporary science has shown to be largely, if not entirely, autoimmune in nature. We are also the most heavily vaccinated country on earth, and there is now a solid body of evidence that not only the MMR vaccine but also the other live-virus vaccines, as well as those containing mercury, aluminum, and other adjuvants, are fully capable of causing autoimmune dysfunction that regularly crosses the blood-brain barrier and causes brain damage. From these experiments, it is only a short step to the inference that autoimmune brain damage is well within the capacity of every vaccine, and indeed an inherent property of the vaccination process itself.

Chapter 7

DEATH

When it happens suddenly and promptly, within hours or days after the vaccination, death is the most obvious example of grievous harm inflicted by vaccines. Yet both the industry and the CDC have evaded taking responsibility for even these most egregious cases, by the simple expedient of giving them an innocuous-sounding name and manipulating the statistics. In addition, it turns out that most vaccine-related deaths do not occur suddenly or promptly. But in either case, whatever the circumstances surrounding them, virtually all deaths following vaccination are dismissed by the same untestable argument that they were coincidental and would have happened anyway.

SUDDEN INFANT DEATH SYNDROME

Sudden deaths in infants have been well-known since ancient times; but until quite recently, most cases were attributed to suffocation, whether intentional or otherwise, and especially to "overlaying" by the parent. With the advent of vaccines in the 1950s, the very real but infrequent possibility of anaphylaxis, an extreme allergic reaction, was clearly recognized and acknowledged; but the clinical impression that sudden death was becoming even more prevalent than that is supported by the increasing attention it began receiving in medical journals and conferences at that time, and indeed ever since.

In a 1972 study, for example, Dr. Alfred Steinschneider concluded that Sudden Infant Death Syndrome, a term of recent coinage, was the result of prolonged apnea;[1] and contemporary work has continued to suggest that many SIDS deaths occur as a result of an apneic episode involving a failure or dysfunction of the breathing reflex, located in the respiratory center of the brain stem.[2] In any case, by the 1980s SIDS had become the leading cause of death in American-born infants up to the age of one year.[3]

The CDC distinguishes three main types of Sudden Unexpected Infant Death, or SUID, in infants less than one year of age:

1. Suffocation, whether accidental or otherwise
2. Sudden Infant Death Syndrome, or SIDS, where the death remains unexplained after a thorough investigation, including a careful history, a postmortem examination of the body, and so forth
3. From unknown cause, where the death is ruled unexplained but an investigation is not done[4]

As is evident from this classification, the only difference between "SIDS" and "Unknown" lies in the thoroughness of medical investigations required to differentiate them, which thus renders both subtypes ripe for manipulation. In 2013, for example, the CDC published the following statistical breakdown for that year:

Reported SUID cases: approx. 3,500
Listed as "SIDS": approx. 1,575 (45%)
Listed as "unknown": approx. 1,085 (31%)
Listed as "suffocation": approx. 880 (24%)[5]

Since 1992, when the American Academy of Pediatrics recommended that infants be put to sleep in the supine position rather than lying prone, as most parents have always preferred, the number of cases listed as SIDS has indeed decreased, but the total number of SUIDs has remained fairly constant at about 3,500–4,000 annually,[6] suggesting that the statistics may have been doctored by simply failing to perform the detailed investigations required for SIDS, thus diagnosing it less often and padding the "unknown" category to make up the difference. In any case, the classification makes no sense, since suffocation is hard to miss, and no other possibilities are contemplated for detailed investigations to identify that might rule out both "SIDS" and "unknown."

Moreover, anaphylaxis is another significant cause of sudden death in infants, as well as older children and adults. It is true that SIDS babies at times die quietly in their sleep, and that anaphylaxis is an allergic phenomenon, typically occurring abruptly within minutes or hours of exposure to the offending substance, and most often presenting with intense and even violent, life-threatening symptoms, most notably choking. Statistically, too, anaphylaxis is classified differently, because it is both familiar enough to be written off as if its cause were known, and rare enough to have been admitted without question and indeed almost eagerly into the vanishingly small official list of adverse reactions to vaccines. But because it is another significant cause of sudden death from vaccines, it would make sense to include it in the same broad category as the others.

The CDC and various pediatric organizations have listed the following as risk factors for SIDS:

1. sleeping in the prone or side position,[7]
2. infection,
3. birth defect,
4. developmental retardation,
5. prematurity or low birth weight, and
6. an older sibling who died of it,

or, in short, just about *anything but* a vaccination.

Given that virtually every child is vaccinated repeatedly in the early months of life, and the peak incidence of SIDS is said to be in the first four months, coinciding with having begun the DTaP, Hib, IPV, Prevnar, Hep B, and rotavirus vaccination series, it is little short of miraculous that the manufacturers have gotten away with keeping vaccines off this list for so long and with so little pushback, a feat rendered all the more impressive by the existence of a considerable body of research linking both SIDS and SUID to vaccination that dates back more than thirty years.

In 1979, for example, the Tennessee Health Department reported four cases of SIDS occurring within 24 hours of their first DPT,[8] while in a much larger retrospective SIDS case study prompted by them, Dr. William Torch found that

6.5%	occurred	within	12 hours	after	a	DPT	shot,
13%	"	"	24 hours	"	"	"	",
26%	"	"	3 days	"	"	"	",
37%	"	"	7 days	"	"	"	",
61%	"	"	14 days	"	"	"	", and
76%	"	"	21 days,[9]				

a strong association that led him to conclude: "DPT may be a major unrecognized cause of sudden infant death, and the risks may outweigh the benefits.

Re-evaluation and possible modification of current policy is indicated by this study."[10]

Further evidence came from Japan, where 57 cases of brain damage and 37 of sudden death were recorded between 1970 and 1974, and were followed by two dramatic SIDS cases in 1975,[11] all of which raised such a storm of protest that the Japanese government decided to postpone all DPT shots until 2 years of age. As the vaccine advocate Dr. James Cherry and his colleagues later conceded, the result of that policy was that "SIDS disappeared when whole-cell and acellular pertussis vaccinations were delayed until 24 months of age."[12]

Yet these same experts never seriously considered adopting such a strategy for the United States, seemingly content that the acellular DTaP was somewhat less toxic, but thereby implicitly acknowledging that both the DTP and the DTaP did in fact cause SIDS, since they found the lower but still ponderable risk of death from the latter sufficiently acceptable to continue the old policy. Officially, neither the CDC nor the bulk of the medical profession has ever admitted that vaccines are in any way responsible for SIDS.

At about the same time, beginning in 1985, even more direct and compelling evidence came to light in Australia. While investigating "cot death," as SIDS is known there, Dr. Viera Scheibner, a senior government research scientist, and Leif Carlsson, an electronics engineer, developed a simple monitoring device that tracked and recorded breathing patterns of young infants from an adjoining room. Designed to sound an alarm if their breathing fell below a certain minimum rate, amplitude, or both, this instrument immediately produced surprising results:

> Parents were reporting alarms while their babies were deeply asleep, often in clusters of 5 to 7 within a 15-minute period. These occurred after the babies were exposed to stress, or a day or two before they developed a cold or cut a tooth. In most cases, they were only breathing shallowly, and soon resumed normal patterns. Some "near-miss" babies who stopped breathing but were found in time and successfully resuscitated showed much higher numbers of alarms than normal, and we realized that they were an important indicator of their general stress level.
>
> Without specifically intending to, we also recorded their breathing before and after they were vaccinated, and the results were extremely significant. We didn't know that the merits of vaccination were being hotly debated at the time. We saw that DPT vaccinations caused babies a lot of stress, in the form of sometimes major flare-ups of shallow breathing or apnea for at least 45–60 days afterward, variable in amplitude but remarkably similar in duration.

> Pediatricians to whom we showed our findings pointed to the arrow indicating the time that the vaccination was given, saying "This is the cause!" and to the abnormal breathing pattern on the ensuing days, saying "This is the effect!" We also learned from parents who monitored a subsequent child after a cot death that most commonly the previous child had died after a DPT injection. We realized that a great number of cot deaths followed DPT injections, and felt we had to address the issue. But when we approached the same pediatricians with these observations and conclusions, we realized that we had touched on a very sensitive area.[13]

Unsurprisingly, as we have since come to expect, the Australian medical community greeted these results with a stony silence, which continues to this day; but as has happened to many other physicians and scientists before and since, both her discoveries and the hostility that greeted them propelled Dr. Scheibner herself into a second career as an activist and committed opponent of mandatory vaccination in any form.

In America, meanwhile, the silence has been equally deafening. After three decades, neither the vaccine establishment nor the vast majority of family physicians and pediatricians have ever seen fit to mention or even notice Scheibner's groundbreaking work, let alone initiate a single study to try to confirm or refute it.

Death as an Inherent Risk of the Vaccination Process

In any case, even if acknowledged and taken seriously, the major contribution of the various DPT vaccines to the tragedy of SIDS still represents only a subset of the general problem of death caused by vaccination, which can occur at any age, from any vaccine, presents clinically in many different ways, and involves a variety of pathological mechanisms. As the most extreme form of brain damage, for example, deaths following an episode of prolonged apnea or simple paralysis of the respiratory center might be thought of as a special case, alongside autism, learning disabilities, and the rest. Many other cases are more complicated than simply dying quietly while asleep, and are preceded by a progressive illness lasting several days, weeks, or even months before ending in death.

I'll begin with a sampling of cases of various types, simply to show that deaths from vaccines are widespread, involve many different pathologies, and are by no means necessarily sudden, or limited to the DPT, DTP, or DTaP. Here is a typical case of SIDS in a newborn baby who died two days after receiving the hepatitis B vaccine, as recounted by his father:

> For the first 12 days of life, Nicholas ate and slept well, like other babies. On the 13th day he was given the Hep B. When I got home from work, he was crying a lot more than usual, even screaming at times, but we'd just taken him for a checkup, and they told us he was big and healthy. We didn't know that vaccines can cause problems. Nicholas cried on and off most of the night. When I went to work the next day, he was still crying, and he continued most of that day and evening too. The next morning my wife found him in his crib, looking as if he'd been dead for several hours. An autopsy showed he had died of SIDS. The pediatrician said he was one of the healthiest babies he'd ever seen.[14]

Because the Hep B is ordinarily given to newborn babies before they leave the hospital, and is thus the very first vaccine they receive, we would expect it to rank high on the list of potentially lethal vaccines. But this boy died of an illness and was in obvious distress for the whole time, to the extent that naming it SIDS, and indeed coining the term to begin with, becomes essentially another way of ignoring the vaccine connection altogether.

The following are two different media accounts of sudden death in the same 12-year-old girl just hours after receiving Gardasil, the HPV vaccine:

> The sudden death of a 12-year-old girl in Waukesha, Wisconsin, hours after receiving the Gardasil vaccine, has shocked the girl's family, and sent out local media asking how this could happen. In a report for *WISN 12 News,* Dr. Geoffrey Swain of the local health department gave the official CDC reply, that severe reactions like this resulting in death are "very rare" for any vaccine, "about 1 in a million." Assuming that that figure is accurate, and taken together with HHS estimates of over 9,000,000 doses per year, that amounts to the government admitting that at least nine girls are killed by the HPV vaccine every year. How many parents know this prior to taking a doctor's advice to administer it?
>
> When the news broke that the girl had died after receiving the HPV vaccine, at least one other parent contacted a local news station to report that her 17-year-old daughter had also had a serious adverse reaction to Gardasil and needed urgent care at a local hospital. A local news affiliate asked, "If it's so rare, what are the odds that another local girl had a similar reaction after getting the shot?"[15]

And here is her mother's first-person account, as reported by another TV station:

> A 12-year-old Wisconsin girl died just hours after she went to the doctor for a sore throat and was given the HPV vaccine while there. Her mother remembers being given a handout about possible side effects. "Thirty minutes later she was trying to sleep, and I kept waking her up." A few hours later, she stepped out briefly to get food, and when she came back she found her daughter on the floor. An experienced EMT, she tried to perform CPR, but to no avail. "The only thing different was that shot," she said; "I wish I'd known more before agreeing to it."[16]

Another death in a very young infant followed soon after the flu vaccine was administered at a routine checkup without his mother's consent when she left the room for a moment:

> Our son Otto was born on August 3, 2014, and received his first vaccines at around two months old. Two weeks later, I took him to the hospital for a checkup after a fall, and he was fine. But when we left we found out that the nurse had given him a flu shot when I left the room, and my dad had gone to the bathroom. I never would've allowed it, but they never asked.
>
> Several days later we found him blue in his crib, with a slight heartbeat. We did CPR and called EMS. He was flown to a different hospital and put on life support, paralyzed from the waist down, with a blood clot in the back of his neck. The doctor said they had ways to get rid of the clot, but they didn't try to remove it before pressuring me to pull the plug on him.
>
> The doctor said he was brain-damaged and should be removed from life support, but we wanted them to give him a chance and do all they could. Still they insisted, and finally the nurse unplugged him, and he passed away in my arms, having just turned three months old.
>
> How many other babies is this happening to? They gave up on him, when I know in my heart that he could've lived. We want them to be held responsible for what they did, and to stop covering up what they're doing to little infants like our son.[17]

With DPT, MMR, and many other common vaccines including multiple components, several of them being administered at the same well-baby visit, and more new ones being added all the time, it has become increasingly difficult to attribute many if not most cases of vaccine-related death to any particular component; and indeed some of the most egregious cases have followed the injection of multiple vaccines simultaneously.

Here is the story of a six-month-old baby boy whose mother delayed his 2-month series to permit his immune system to begin developing on its own, evidently as a punishment for which the boy was injected with no fewer than 13 different vaccines simultaneously without her permission:

> When her son was six months old, his mother took him in for a round of vaccinations to a clinic in Fort Worth, Texas. She had delayed giving him his two-month shots to allow his immune system to develop a bit more, but the pediatrician was telling her how important vaccinations were, and how many children died without them in Africa.
>
> Without her knowledge or consent, the boy received a total of 13 different vaccines that day, including two doses of DTaP, Hepatitis B, Polio, three oral Rotavirus, and a Pneumococcus, all combined into three shots and a single oral cocktail; it took the nurses half an hour to prepare them. The pediatrician said that the boy was perfectly healthy and showed above-average strength in his stomach and legs.
>
> When she brought him home that day he was twitching a lot, extremely cranky, no longer making eye contact, and had a red knot on his leg at the injection site. Five days later he died, while sleeping on his mother's chest.[18]

Once again, the SIDS label seems totally inadequate as a description of the event, let alone an explanation; as in the Gardasil case, this boy died quietly in his sleep, but only after several days of symptoms, notably twitching, extreme irritability, and loss of eye contact, suggesting ongoing brain damage.

Here is another even more ghastly example—if that is possible—once again involving a young infant who died after receiving 8 vaccines at once:

> Crystal Downing and her husband are distraught from the death of their infant son after being vaccinated. He died in his sleep and was taken to the hospital afterwards. His death was ruled a SIDS, but the couple was not allowed to take his body home until an autopsy was performed.
>
> After numerous phone calls were made and several weeks had gone by without receiving any notice, they were finally told they could not view his remains before the cremation, even to say goodbye; and as of today, 16 months later, they have still not received the autopsy report. They found out that he had been given 8 vaccines that day, including one not approved for someone his age, as well as an extra dose of Hep B that he should not have received until later on.[19]

How well aware the industry itself has always been that its products have the power to kill, whether quickly or slowly, is attested to in this secret memo from GlaxoSmithKline, which was subpoenaed by an Italian court and leaked to the press by a company employee:

> A confidential GlaxoSmithKline document recently leaked to the press exposed that within a two-year period, a total of 36 infants died after receiving the 6-in-1 vaccine, Infanrix Hexa (DTaP, Hep B, Hib, IPV). According to the website that first reported the news, the 1271-page document detailed a total of 1,742 reports of adverse reactions between October 23, 2009, and October 22, 2011, including 503 serious adverse reactions and 36 deaths. The website further stated:
>
> We also found data for 37 others, bringing the total to at least 73 deaths since the launch of the vaccine in 2000, and this applies only to sudden death. Finally, since very few adverse reactions to vaccines are actually reported, anywhere from 1% to 10%, the actual number of deaths is probably much higher.[20]

The same GSK document was later published by the National Library of Medicine, an analysis of which shows that the number of deaths in the first 10 days after vaccination was vastly greater than that in the next 10 days, thus clearly implicating the vaccine and ruling out the manufacturer's long-standing insistence that the deaths were simply due to SIDS (i.e., what would have been expected under normal circumstances and therefore coincidental).

> If one looks at the deaths in the first 10 days after administration of vaccine and compares [them] to the deaths in the next 10 days, it is clear that 97% of deaths (65) in the infants below 1 year occurred in the first ten days, and only 3% (2) occurred in the next ten days. Had the deaths been coincidental SIDS deaths unrelated to vaccination, the numbers of deaths should have been the same for both ten-day periods. Similarly in children older than one year, seven deaths, or 87.5%, occurred in the first ten days, and one, or 12.5%, occurred in the next ten days.[21]

In addition, the extensive underreporting of adverse reactions, amounting to about 1% of the true figure, according to Dr. Kessler, or 10% by the more parsimonious CDC estimate, prompted me to look at eyewitness reports of SIDS and various other deaths and serious injuries that have been submitted by email to the Think Twice Global Vaccine Institute, a website with a long and distinguished history of publishing and advocacy on behalf of the vaccine-injured. A brief sampling follows.

MMR

"My dear friend lost her 15-month-old daughter two weeks after her MMR. She was healthy and showed no sign of illness, yet died suddenly in her sleep one afternoon. The postmortem revealed a viral infection and traces of pneumonia, but her mother and I find it very hard to believe that the vaccine wasn't to blame."[22]

MMR

"Ten days after MMR was injected into our daughter, she was dead; she was only 17 months old. We were told to expect a mild reaction after ten days. We're dealing with government-sanctioned corporate profiteering and killing at taxpayers' expense."[23]

Hib

"My daughter was born healthy and progressing great. Then I got a mail reminder that she was due for her shots. I made an appointment and she got them. One week later she was dead. The autopsy report came back as '*Haemophilus influenzae.*' She was not ill in any way, but now she's dead. They keep saying it can't happen, but what more proof do they need?"[24]

Hib

"A child I cared for recently died at 15 months of age from a reaction to the Hib vaccine. It seemed like SIDS because he died in his sleep."[25]

Pneumococcus

"I had a baby that was perfectly healthy, happy, and OK until she got her Prevnar vaccine. Thirty hours later she's in the hospital having seizures that they can't stop. You're not going to tell me it's not related to the vaccine somehow." [This child slipped into and out of coma for 45 days, shaking with tremors most of the time, until she died.][26]

Influenza

"In November my wife had a flu shot for the first time. For the next five days, she had flu-like symptoms; then she felt better and seemed back to normal for two days. But the next day she was in bed again, complaining about me trying to wake her, agitated, and vociferous: most unusual. Within an hour, her condition worsened, and I called the doctor, who hospitalized her immediately. She died there 3 weeks later, without her doctors finding any cause; the postmortem stated that she had died from a reaction to the flu vaccine."[27]

Influenza

"My husband's aunt, who was very healthy, got a flu shot and became ill afterward for about 4 weeks, never improving until she died."[28]

Influenza

"One of our patients died three days after a routine flu shot. A few days later we read the lovely lady's obituary, in which her death was not reported as a reaction to the vaccine."[29]

Chicken pox

"A healthy 18-month-old boy with no history of allergy or adverse vaccine reaction was admitted to the ICU four days after his chicken pox shot with a low platelet count and bleeding from the mouth. He died two days later from a cerebral hemorrhage."[30]

Oral polio

"Four months ago my son was given the polio vaccine without my knowledge; I would never have agreed to it. He changed from that day, with high-pitched screaming, smelly stools, nonstop crying, difficulty breathing, high fever, and lethargy. He lost weight, and his development ceased. My wife was six months pregnant. About a week after my son's vaccination, she began having headaches, weakness, tiredness, and loss of balance, everything pointing to polio infection. Then she had to go to the hospital because of something wrong with the pregnancy, and she lost the baby. I tried to test for polio and to find the cause of this tragic series of events, but the medical profession was extremely unhelpful. They just laughed at me. I'll never know why our son stopped growing and developing, or why we lost our daughter. The only thing I'm sure about is that the precursor of these events was the polio vaccine."[31]

Having already cited fatal reactions to DPT, hepatitis B, and the HPV vaccine, I need not add to them here. I haven't yet seen any cases of death reported after the shingles or rotavirus vaccines, nor have I tried to analyze the DPT and MMR cases to assign them to one specific component. But even this small sampling is more than sufficient to establish that the demographic of vaccine-related deaths is a heterogeneous one that includes

1. newborns, infants, children, adolescents, and more than a few adults;
2. a number of different vaccines and combinations thereof, with very few if any exceptions; and
3. a variety of clinical and pathological syndromes and presentations, ranging from dying quietly while asleep without any previous symptoms, to definite illnesses, many of an autoimmune type, and lasting from several days to several weeks, with dyspnea and choking, brain damage, clotting and hemorrhagic phenomena, to name only a few of the possibilities.

I would add to these established facts the significant weight of evidence that the risk of death is more or less directly proportional to the number of vaccine components administered at the same clinic visit, a hypothesis that also tallies very closely with the questions, doubts, anxieties, intuitions, hunches, and "gut feelings" expressed by most new parents who seek my advice on how best to vaccinate their kids.

Evidently, Dr. Wakefield also felt the same way in 1998, when even his modest recommendation that the three components of the MMR vaccine be administered separately so alarmed and infuriated the CDC and the medical community on both sides of the pond that he was cashiered in disgrace from his hospital post, lost his license to practice, and experienced the deliberate and systematic ruining of his reputation. Perhaps even more to the point, our propensity to look no further than the specific effects of specific vaccines distracts us from being curious about the effect of the vaccination process *per se,* and thus gives the CDC and the vaccine manufacturers the green light to pile on as many more new vaccines as they like, without ever having to consider what every thoughtful parent appropriately fears, and on some level intuitively knows, that the crucial variable is the total number of vaccine events, whether tallied simultaneously at the same visit, or cumulatively over the patient's lifetime.

In its extreme form, unrestrained by even the pretense of a comprehensive investigation into how vaccines really act, this enthusiastic salesmanship for the vaccine concept is the trademark contribution of Paul Offit, MD, who not only profits extravagantly from RotaTeq, the rotavirus vaccine that he developed and patented, but also serves on the ACIP and helps formulate its mandates and recommendations for national vaccine policy. He once famously boasted that the newborn infant could easily tolerate and indeed benefit from 10,000 vaccines simultaneously,[32] a bravado that has prompted many calls for him to show good faith by volunteering his own body to support that claim.

In addition, many experimental vaccines are first tested in Third World countries with even looser standards and enforcement than our own, as in this sensational news story from Argentina, where a pneumococcal vaccine caused 14 deaths in babies who received it after only a sham of parental consent, obtained by bullying and intimidation:

> GlaxoSmithKline Argentina was fined 400,000 pesos by Judge Marcelo Aguinsky following a report issued by the National Administration of Medicine, Food and Technology for irregularities during lab vaccine trials conducted between 2007 and 2008 that allegedly killed 14 babies. Two doctors were also fined 300,000 pesos each for experimentation upon human beings with nothing but falsified parental authorizations.
>
> Pediatrician Ana Marchese, who reported the case to the Argentine Federation of Health Professionals, was working at the Eva Perón Public Children's Hospital in Santiago del Estero when the studies were conducted, and said this morning on AM radio that "These doctors took advantage of illiterate parents by pressuring them into signing these 28-page consent forms." Colombia and Panama were also chosen by GSK as staging grounds for trials of the vaccine.[33]

In another equally scandalous affair, two babies were killed and 37 hospitalized in rural Mexico when a combination of three vaccines were given to 52 babies for a casualty rate of 75%:

> The latest vaccine tragedy has killed two babies in La Pimienta, Mexico, and sent 37 more to the hospital with serious reactions, with "14 in serious condition, 22 stable, and one critical," the Chiapas Health Secretariat said on Latino.FoxNews.com. What is especially alarming is that only 52 children were vaccinated, and 75% of them are dead or hospitalized.

> The Tuberculosis, Rotavirus and Hepatitis B vaccines were administered by the Mexican Social Security Institute, or IMSS, which confirmed the deadly reactions. According to Fox News Latino, IMSS has suspended the vaccines pending the outcome of an investigation. According to the mainstream media in the US, vaccines never harm anyone and are perfectly safe to inject into children in unlimited quantities. This denialism is rampant across the corporate-controlled media, which refuse to acknowledge the truth that vaccines kill and injure children on a regular basis.[34]

Similarly unethical and ultimately lethal trials were conducted by the William & Melinda Gates Foundation and the WHO in tribal areas of India, where 16,000 girls, aged 9 to 15, received Merck's Gardasil HPV vaccine, as a result of which hundreds developed seizures, premature menstruation, and other illnesses, and 5 died, while 14,000 received Cervarix, the GlaxoSmithKline version, and 2 died.[35] An investigation by the Indian Supreme Court revealed that the children were living in hostels while at school, and that consent was given for the trials by hostel wardens without their parents' knowledge, as a result of which the Gates Foundation and WHO are being sued by the Indian Government and have been widely accused of unethical conduct by doctors and politicians alike.[36]

In all of these cases, the Gates Foundation and WHO have continued to insist that the illnesses and deaths are coincidental and unrelated to the vaccinations. What these scandals make clear is that death from a vaccination is simply the most extreme possibility, at the far end of the whole spectrum of possible adverse reactions, that it involves *all* vaccines, and is thus an inherent risk of the vaccination process *per se.*

THE "SHAKEN-BABY SYNDROME"

Another significant cause of underreporting is the tendency of some pediatricians and judges, no doubt partly in response to the discovery of "shaken-baby syndrome" and signs of apparent traumatic brain injury in autopsied victims of infant and child abuse, to assume that SIDS deaths involving brain hemorrhage are due to child abuse, and to convict and imprison parents and other caregivers on that inference, without ever considering recent vaccinations as potentially important contributory evidence.

In an infamous 1997 case from Florida, a father was convicted of child abuse of his 10-week-old son and sentenced to life in prison, even though the medical examiner's testimony that convicted him had been falsified in several key respects,[37] while my own review of the baby's medical records, corroborated by that of several other physicians, found them entirely consistent with the possibility of an encephalopathic reaction to the combined DTaP, Hib, OPV, and Hep B vaccines, all of which he had received simultaneously only a few days earlier.[38] In 2004, after serving over six years in the State Penitentiary, the father was finally exonerated and released, and his accuser given a harsh sentence for his misconduct, which allowed the Court to escape having to implicate the vaccinations or rule on the actual cause of death.[39]

In any case, the outcry occasioned by the imprisonment of so many parents and caregivers has belatedly prompted a number of physicians to reconsider the validity of the syndrome itself. To give just one example, Michael Innis, MD, a retired British hematologist, wrote an article to the effect that the so-called "shaken-baby syndrome" is essentially an inaccurate diagnosis, and that very many, if not all, such cases represent an autoimmune disturbance of the clotting mechanism, involving a defect of vitamin C metabolism, and implicating vaccines and other common antigens as well:

> A pediatric consultant has testified in the trial of a child minder charged with assaulting a baby that the baby's injuries were caused by shaking. Parents and caregivers are often falsely accused of having inflicted unexplained bruises, fractures, retinal and subdural hemorrhages with "ischemic encephalopathy," the alleged signs of physical abuse, a condition named "shaken-baby syndrome" in 1971. These features can also be an autoimmune reaction which destroys the insulin-producing cells of the pancreas, as evidenced by hyperglycemia in these children, which the doctors overlooked.
>
> When vaccinated children with these conditions were investigated, damaged beta-cells were found in the pancreas, resulting in hypoinsulinemia, inhibited cellular uptake of vitamins C and K, and liver dysfunction, hemorrhages, and fractures. These are autoimmune responses in genetically susceptible individuals, commonly to mandated vaccines, or viral, bacterial, and parasitic infections. Until the medical profession realizes that shaken-baby syndrome is a fabricated diagnosis lacking any scientific evidence, they will continue to accuse innocent people falsely and send hundreds of them to prison.[40]

Finally, simply to underline the fact that death from vaccinations is an ever-present possibility, I looked at the 92 cases of Vaccine Court awards for vaccine injuries, as listed by the US Department of Justice, for the quarter between November 16, 2014, and February 15, 2015. There were a total of 6 deaths:

1 death:	Hepatitis A	10 months
1 death:	DTaP, Hib, IPV, pneumo	8 years, 2 months
4 deaths:	Influenza:	
	1 Guillain-Barré syndrome	2 years, 10 months
	1 Guillain-Barré syndrome	1 year, 9 months
	1 cardiomyopathy	1 year, 4 months
	1 "as a result of injuries"	1 year, 5 months[41]

The striking preponderance of deaths from the flu vaccine, the coincidence of the Guillain-Barré syndrome causing two of them, and the same vaccine prompting awards in an amazingly large number of the nonlethal cases as well, aroused my curiosity still further, since it corroborated my sense that death often represents nothing more than an extreme version along the continuum of neurological and other systemic injury. I found the following:

Out of a total of 92 such awards,

- Sixty-eight cases (73.9%) followed the flu vaccine given alone;
- Six cases (6.5%) followed the flu vaccine given with others, for a total of seventy-four cases (80.4%) involving the flu vaccine;
- Twenty cases (21.7%) following the flu vaccine alone or with others involved CNS diagnoses other than Guillain-Barré syndrome, namely, encephalitis, myelitis, polyneuropathy, neuralgia, and myositis; several involved GBS as well;
- Fifty-one cases (55.4%) received awards for GBS;
- Forty-five of these (48.9%) were for the flu vaccine given alone; and
- Three of these (3.2%) were for the flu vaccine given together with others.[42]

I shall say more about the flu vaccine in a later chapter. For now, I will simply repeat that death represents only the severest form of vaccine injury; that it most often involves some form of brain and/or neurological damage, but can occur with almost any kind of systemic pathology, and after receiving virtually any vaccine. In spite of all the underreporting, all the difficulties in obtaining reliable statistics, and for all the reasons previously discussed, it is evident that the numbers killed in this fashion are quite substantial, although largely denied and carefully hidden by both the industry and the CDC, and still unacknowledged by the vast majority of the medical profession.

It seems only fitting to give the last word on this subject to Barbara Loe Fisher, author of *DPT: a Shot in the Dark,* cofounder of NVIC, and mother of a brain-injured son, who has advocated tirelessly for vaccine-injured children and their parents for the past thirty-five years, and knows what is really happening out there probably better than any other living soul:

> Memorial Day is for remembering those who have fought and died to defend America and preserve our civil liberties. So every Memorial Day I remember the children who have died after receiving mandated vaccines, and honor the parents who grieve for them.
>
> From the beginning, death has always been a consequence of vaccination. In 1933, two infants died within minutes of their pertussis shot. In 1946, twins died suddenly within 24 hours of their second DPT shot. Since 1986, the Government has awarded over $2 billion in compensation for deaths and injuries caused by vaccines.
>
> A nation which spends more per capita on healthcare and requires their children to get more vaccines than any other should have one of the best infant mortality rates, not one of the worst. When healthy babies die shortly after their vaccinations, parents legitimately ask whether vaccines did it, and are met with quick denials by doctors and public health officials.
>
> Their death certificates typically list SIDS as the cause, which means that no specific symptoms or reason for death could be found. Yet most babies dying after their shots are not found dead in their cribs without any symptoms, but rather have suffered for days with high fever, collapse, screaming, arching of the back, diarrhea, and the like, which their pediatricians often dismiss as unimportant. Others suffer mental and physical deterioration that gets worse after each shot until they are found dead in the crib. The inconvenient truth remains that there are more full-term babies dying before their first birthday than in most developed nations of the world.[43]

SUMMARY

The official government system for classifying infant deaths is completely inadequate and indeed seems explicitly designed to rule out any possibility of vaccines playing a significant causal role. In the first place, only sudden deaths are included, whereas deaths following vaccination can occur at any time within hours, days, months, or even years later, and often involve variable periods of illness preceding them.

In the second place, there are only three recognized categories: (1) suffocation, which is rare, (2) SIDS, in which death remains unexplained even after thorough medical and laboratory examination, and vaccination is thus ruled out by definition (since in that case it would no longer be unexplained), and (3) "unknown," which is identical to SIDS, except that such examinations are not done. And finally, anaphylaxis is not included, even though if not precisely because it is known and accepted to be caused by vaccines.

In reality, deaths following vaccination and clearly traceable to it on obvious clinical grounds are widespread, take many forms, and can occur after any vaccine. For all of these reasons, the whole classification, and especially the terms "Sudden Unexpected Infant Death," or SUID, and "Sudden Infant Death Syndrome," or SIDS, should be abandoned, for the simple reason that they are defined in such a way as to obscure the mere possibility of a link to any vaccine.

Chapter 8

THE VACCINE COURT

THE NATIONAL CHILDHOOD VACCINE INJURY ACT

In 1986, in response to the sadness and outrage of the unprecedented numbers of parents whose children had died or suffered brain damage after being vaccinated, and the considerable public outcry on their behalf, Congress passed the National Childhood Vaccine Injury Act. The wording of the statute was accordingly populist in tone, outwardly sympathetic to the needs of these devastated families, and promised speedy and efficient relief, as the distinguished legal scholar and historian Mary Holland has pointed out: "The Law established the Vaccine Injury Compensation Program to compensate 'vaccine-related injury or death.' In it Congress asserted that its purpose was *'to establish a no-fault program under which awards can be made to the vaccine-injured quickly, easily, and with certainty and generosity.'*"[1]

The Act created two new federal initiatives, which are administered separately and are technically independent of each other, but share the same basic principles and adhere to virtually identical standards and guidelines for determining whether or not adverse reactions are vaccine-related, namely,

1. the Vaccine Adverse Events Reporting System, or VAERS, a database for government agencies, health providers, and parents to report deaths and injuries following vaccinations, and possibly caused by them
2. the Vaccine Injury Compensation Program, or VICP, a no-fault system for prompt settlement of valid legal claims of vaccine injury as an alternative to litigation

The less edifying backstory emerged from the large number of successful damage claims for DPT encephalopathy, which had established that vaccine manufacturers were indeed liable and obliged to pay for the injuries and ruined lives they had caused, just like any other company, a bedrock principle dating back to the origins of the common law. To avoid the expense and bad publicity of such litigation in the future, Big Pharma simply threatened to stop making vaccines altogether unless Congress agreed to exempt them from the same level of responsibility that every other industry is required to assume.

It is a testament to the power, standing, and influence of the drug industry in American society that, thanks to these machinations, the promised remedy of easy, swift, and generous remuneration of the victims was swiftly transformed into its exact opposite, an adversarial "Vaccine Court" process that was effectively rigged against them, by cementing in place the industry's minimal safety standards that had created the problem in the first place, as a result of which no claimants receive so much as an apology, and vanishingly few win significant relief.

THE VAERS REPORTING SYSTEM

Although its mission statement sounds objective and value-neutral in simply providing a mechanism for parents to report suspected adverse events, the VAERS is the logical starting point for the VICP as well, because its criteria for deciding whether or not a bad outcome is vaccine-related also play a decisive role in the quasi-judicial process by which the Vaccine Court rules for or against the damage claims submitted to it.

Under joint supervision of the FDA and the CDC, the Vaccine Adverse Events Reporting System was ostensibly developed as a tool for post-marketing surveillance, to augment and fine-tune the safety studies that the manufacturers were required to conduct and obtain FDA approval for before making each vaccine widely available to the general public. As outlined on the CDC website, it sounds like an innocuous and indeed eminently sensible refinement:

> Licensure requires extensive evaluation of the vaccine's safety and efficacy. First, laboratory and animal studies are performed. Then vaccines are tested in small groups of adult volunteers. Finally, large-scale clinical trials, *usually randomized and placebo-controlled,* measure protective efficacy and the rates of the more common adverse events. *The control groups who do not receive the vaccine are critical to distinguishing between vaccine-related events and those unrelated to the vaccine that occur spontaneously in the study population.*

> Post-marketing surveillance is a necessary component of vaccine safety monitoring. Due to the relatively small number of patients studied before licensing, rarer side-effects that only occur in subgroups of the population not significantly represented in pre-marketing studies, such as neonates, pregnant women, and immunosuppressed patients, or that occur only with chronic or repeated exposure to a vaccine antigen or component, may not be revealed until the vaccine is licensed to the general public. Increasingly, manufacturers are being asked to conduct "Phase IV" post-licensure trials as a precondition of licensure. [Italics mine: R. M.][2]

On its face, the document gives every appearance of conscientiously serving the public good, by looking for adverse reactions that might have been missed in the safety trials, as well as conveying the definite impression that VAERS reports from parents and providers will be welcomed and indeed eagerly solicited. The reality, however, could hardly be more different.

In the first place, the professed commitment to placebo-controlled trials is a bald-faced lie. As we saw, the industry's misnamed "placebo-control groups" are actually given other vaccines, or the adjuvant alone, not the inert placebo that is here specified, and widely accepted as the proper way to distinguish between vaccine-related events and those occurring randomly by chance.

In the second place, just as with the premarketing safety trials, the criteria for determining that events are vaccine-caused rather than merely coincidental are so stringent that in practice they are seldom satisfied:

SIDE EFFECTS AFTER VACCINATION: TEMPORAL VS. CAUSAL ASSOCIATIONS[3]

An adverse event can be causally attributed to a vaccine if

1. the exact chronology of vaccination and adverse event onset is known;
2. the adverse event corresponds to those previously associated with a particular vaccine;
3. the event conforms to a specific clinical syndrome whose association with vaccination has strong biological plausibility (e.g., anaphylaxis);
4. a laboratory result confirms the association (e.g., isolation of vaccine-strain virus from the patient);

5. the event recurs on re-administration of the vaccine ("positive-rechallenge"); and
6. a controlled clinical trial or epidemiologic study shows greater risk of the specific adverse event in vaccinated than in unvaccinated control groups.

Let us consider these points one by one.

Chronology

Although seemingly straightforward and noncontroversial, precise chronology is often misleading and difficult to obtain in reality, because the chronic, autoimmune diseases that are prominent among the adverse effects most commonly reported tend to develop slowly and insidiously, and are thus automatically ruled out from the start. A perfect example was the case I cited earlier of renal failure following an MMR vaccine, which began as a nondescript flu-like illness fully 2 weeks after the shot, and manifested as the full-blown nephrotic syndrome only 6 weeks later. In practice, the term "exact chronology" is employed simply to exclude these vague, subclinical beginnings, and is almost always restricted to something very acute and dramatic that develops very soon after receiving the vaccine, such as anaphylaxis, where the link is so blatant that even the CDC has never seen fit to deny or question it, and indeed has all but trumpeted it as evidence of its good faith.

Only Reactions Already Described

The second requirement, which is that adverse events must correspond to clinical entities already described, is even more restrictive:

1. by ruling out the possibility of discovering a new complication not previously identified, even though the stated purpose of conducting post-marketing surveillance was precisely that;
2. by limiting the investigation to specific effects of specific vaccines, and overlooking nonspecific effects of the vaccination process itself, no matter which vaccine it happens to be.

"Biologically Plausible"

I confess to having not the slightest idea what is meant by "biological plausibility," other than yet another reason for disqualifying chronic, autoimmune illnesses from consideration, since the question why a previously healthy organism would begin to attack and destroy its own tissues has never been answered satisfactorily, and thus might well be regarded as automatically implausible in that sense.

Laboratory Confirmation

This one is the most interesting, because it's a sword that cuts both ways. In most instances, laboratory confirmation seems impractical and inconvenient, and indeed is rarely performed; it is invoked as yet another obstacle for discrediting reports of adverse effects not previously identified. Nobody bothers to draw blood for anaphylaxis because it's already on the list, or to look for autoantibodies in cases of SIDS, which has already been predefined as a coincidence unrelated to vaccines.

On the other hand, Dr. Wakefield's work was rightly perceived as threatening, because unequivocal and indeed irrefutable laboratory confirmation was precisely what it *did* provide for the first time. His elegant biopsy specimens demonstrated antibodies to the measles virus and lesions of autoimmune inflammatory bowel disease in the lymphoid aggregates of his autistic patients' intestinal tracts. With no way to refute these findings, the industry and the CDC saw no option but to vilify and destroy him personally.

So yes, I'm all for laboratory confirmation, if it is applicable, and indicates something worth measuring. With autoimmunity as possibly the underlying mechanism by which vaccines do everything they do, good and bad alike, why not screen children for evidence of it in the form of C-reactive protein, erythrocyte sedimentation rate (ESR), antinuclear antibodies (ANA), and perhaps other typical markers at suitable intervals after their vaccinations? Although by no means infallible, and possibly subject to both false positives and negatives, just as in clinical medicine, it would nevertheless be a simple, interesting, and inexpensive test of that hypothesis, whether or not those testing positive actually develop symptoms at the time.

The "Positive-Rechallenge" Test

More than just impractical and counterproductive, this criterion borders on the fiendish, because administering another dose of the same vaccine that resulted in an adverse reaction is highly likely to provoke an even worse result the next time, as Barbara Loe Fisher's book, Yehuda Shoenfeld's meticulous research, and my own clinical experience all bear witness to, while the adolescent girls who die of their HPV or flu shots, or the infants who die of SIDS after their DTaP or Hep B, are unfortunately already dead and therefore sadly unavailable for further doses.

Confirmation by Randomized Controlled Trial

This final criterion is pure and simple hypocrisy, because confirmation of the vaccine linkage by a randomized, placebo-controlled clinical trial is precisely what the CDC and the industry should have done in the premarketing phase, and steadfastly refused to do; so they shouldn't be allowed to get away with listing it as yet another reason for disqualification after the fact, despite having themselves rejected it on principle long before.

REPORTABLE EVENTS FOLLOWING VACCINATION

As a result of all of these restrictions, VAERS reports of injury and VICP claims of damage will be certified as vaccine-related if and only if they conform to the same impossibly rigid standards as those of the premarketing safety trials we have already discussed:

Reportable Events Following Vaccination:[4]

Vaccine or Toxoid	Event and interval post-vaccination	
Tetanus toxoid	Anaphylaxis or anaphylactic shock Brachial neuritis Any acute complications or sequelae of the above, including death	7 days 28 days N/A
Pertussis	Anaphylaxis or anaphylactic shock Encephalitis or encephalopathy Any acute complications or sequelae of the above, including death Events described in package insert as a contraindication to additional doses	7 days 7 days N/A see insert

MMR	Anaphylaxis or anaphylactic shock Encephalitis or encephalopathy Any acute complications or sequelae of the above, including death Events described in package insert as a contra-indication to additional doses	7 days 15 days N/A see insert
Rubella	Chronic arthritis Any acute complications or sequelae of the above, including death Events described in package insert as a contraindication to additional doses	42 days N/A see insert
Measles	Thrombocytopenic purpura Vaccine-strain measles in immunodeficient recipient Any acute complications or sequelae of the above, including death Events described in package insert as a contraindication to additional doses	7–30 days 6 months N/A see insert
Oral polio (OPV)	Paralytic polio: -in immunocompetent recipient -in immunodeficient recipient -in community contact Vaccine-strain polio (same 3 types:) Any acute complications or sequelae of the above, including death Events described in package insert as a contraindication to additional doses	 30 days 6 months N/A same N/A see insert
Injectable polio (IPV)	Anaphylaxis or anaphylactic shock Any acute complications or sequelae of the above, including death Events described in package insert as a contraindication to additional doses	7 days N/A see insert
Hepatitis B	Anaphylaxis or anaphylactic shock Any acute complications or sequelae of the above, including death Events described in package insert as a contraindication to additional doses	7 days N/A see insert

Hib	Events described in package insert as a contraindication to additional doses	see insert
Varicella	Events described in package insert as a contraindication to additional doses	see insert
Rotavirus	Events described in package insert as a contraindication to additional doses	see insert
Pneumococcal conjugate	Events described in package insert as a contraindication to additional doses	see insert
Hepatitis A	Events described in package insert as a contraindication to additional doses	see insert
Influenza, trivalent inactivated	Events described in package insert as a contraindication to additional doses	see insert
Influenza, live attenuated	Events described in package insert as a contraindication to additional doses	see insert
Meningococcal conjugate	Events described in package insert as a contraindication to additional doses	see insert
HPV, bivalent or quadrivalent	Events described in package insert as a contraindication to additional doses	see insert

Far from its stated purpose of expanding the list to include whatever else is out there, the practical effect is precisely the opposite, to ensure that most reports originating from the general public that somebody was killed or maimed after being vaccinated will be rejected, in precisely the same way and for precisely the same reasons that unsolicited reports of adverse reactions in the manufacturers' safety trials were dismissed as coincidental by the lead investigator. *That* degree of consistency is surely no coincidence.

The Vaccine Injury Table used by the VICP is essentially identical to the VAERS Table of Reportable Events, but even more restrictive about the maximum time limit allowed between the vaccine and the first sign of injury.[5] Only the very few and vanishingly rare adverse reactions that are deemed "reportable" to the VAERS system are likely to win a substantial claim of damages in the Vaccine Court.

Whether we accept the CDC's estimate of only 10% of adverse events being reported, or the former FDA Commissioner David Kessler's figure of 1%, even a cursory glance at the list makes it easy to understand why so few parents of victims ever bother to file a claim or even report an injury, when the system that allegedly seeks and values their participation is stacked against them so heavily that their stories will seldom be believed or taken seriously.

FILING A VAERS REPORT

Above and beyond these built-in obstacles and formal impediments, but wholly consistent with them, is the frustrating ordeal that many parents actually experience when they do try to report an injury. Here is an excerpt from the narrative of a woman whose daughter suffered a grand mal seizure hours after a TdaP booster:

> My daughter's vaccine injury occurred within 3 hours of being given the Tdap vaccine; she had a grand mal seizure, fell off the bed, hit her head, and stopped breathing while I held her head in my hands. Thankfully, she was resuscitated, and we went to the hospital in an ambulance. I called our family doctor, who had given her the vaccine, and said I wanted her reaction reported to VAERS as a vaccine injury.
>
> We went to the hospital, and I told them what had happened; they knew it was a vaccine injury. Months later, it still hadn't been reported, and I called my doctor to ask why. The office staff said, we didn't have to report it, because you didn't bring her back here. I said, I didn't bring her there because she stopped breathing, and we went to the hospital in an ambulance. They said, then the *hospital* should have reported it.
>
> So I called the hospital, and they said, we didn't give the vaccine; the *physician* should have reported it. I called the VAERS office and asked whose responsibility it is to report vaccine injuries. I told her the situation; she said, *either one* should have reported it. I said, isn't that mandatory? She said yes. I asked, what are the consequences if physicians fail to report? She said, *none.* But if there aren't any consequences, that's a suggestion, not a law.[6]

In a similar vein, here is what happened when a father tried to report the death of his newborn daughter after her second Hep B shot:

> My daughter Lyla Rose died at 5 weeks of age, shortly after receiving a Hepatitis B booster shot. She was lively and alert, and gazed into my eyes with the innocence and wonder of a newborn child; she was never ill before that shot.

At her final feeding afterwards, she was agitated and feisty, and then fell asleep and didn't wake up. The autopsy ruled out choking; brain swelling was the only finding. The doctors said it must be SIDS, a catch-all diagnosis for unexplainable childhood death. My wife and I agonized over what we might have missed or could have done, but I kept returning to the obvious medical event that preceded her death. The doctors said the vaccine was safe, but on searching the Internet I found disturbing evidence of adverse reactions to it.

I attended a Hep B Vaccine Safety Forum at the Institute of Medicine, at which scientists presented cases of nervous system damage, like MS, while the FDA presented a study from its VAERS System, which showed only 19 neonatal deaths since 1991 related to the vaccine, data I found to be completely deceptive. Lyla Rose died within the sample period, and wasn't even counted; the New York City Coroner called VAERS to report her death, and no one ever returned his call. What kind of reporting system doesn't return the calls of the New York City Medical Examiner? How many other reports are ignored? I listened in amazement as CDC officials and Merck's head of Vaccine Safety made disparaging comments about any possible risk from the vaccine, despite the evidence just presented.

As a financial consultant trained in econometrics, I can tell you that the VAERS study is an illegitimate data set from which no conclusions about large populations can be made. There are 17,000 reports of adverse reactions to Hep B vaccine in the 1996–97 raw data alone. If VAERS doesn't even return the Medical Examiner's call, how many other deaths and injuries go unreported? My impression is that Merck and the CDC don't know or want to know how many babies are being killed or injured by vaccines. If there were 17,000 reports of a new, dangerous disease in an 18-month period, the CDC would be all over it. But there are 17,000 reports of adverse reactions to a vaccine, and they dismiss them as coincidence.[7]

As both stories make clear, the problem with the VAERS system is not merely that the public is unaware of its existence,

1. because doctors and nurses are required by law to report vaccine injuries, and regularly neglect to do so;
2. because even when the medical examiner of the City of New York files a report, it gets lost or dismissed; and
3. because SIDS, for example, has already been defined in advance as a death without known cause, and will therefore not be counted, no matter who reports it, or how soon after the vaccination it occurs.

An extensive, firsthand experience of the same problem is provided by this compelling online testimony of a veteran emergency room nurse who cares for acute vaccine injuries on a regular basis. She found no other venue for expressing her anger at the systematic cover-up by her colleagues and superiors, and prudently chose to remain anonymous, no doubt justly fearing disciplinary action or worse for daring to speak out about it:

> As an ER nurse, I've seen the cover-up. Where do kids go when they have a vaccine reaction? They go to the ER; they come to me. I can't say how many reactions I've seen over the years. It has to be in the hundreds, sometimes one or two cases in a single shift, every shift, for weeks. Then a lull for a week or two, then another case every night for a couple of weeks: this is common.
>
> Say the child comes in with 105° fever, seizures, lethargy, and can't wake up, spasms, or screaming that won't stop. My first question is, if they're current on their shots, to see how recently they were vaccinated, to decide if it's a vaccine reaction. Too often the parents say, "Yes, the pediatrician gave the vaccines this morning, and said they were in perfect health!" If I had a dollar for every time I've heard that, I could fly to Europe for free.
>
> But here's the most disturbing part. For all these cases, I've never seen any other nurse or doctor report them to VAERS. I've served in many states, with over a hundred doctors and at least 300–400 nurses, in hospitals big and small. When I say never, I mean NEVER. I sit at the Nurses' Station filling out VAERS reports to make sure they see me doing it. The other nurses say, "I've never done that," or "I didn't know we could do that," or ask, "What is VAERS?" From the doctors, total silence, absolute refusal to talk about it.
>
> The CDC and HHS admit they hear about 1/10th of the actual number of injuries; but from my experience, I'd say it's more like 1/1000th of the reality. I've also seen deliberate omissions and falsifications of medical records by doctors, after the child was vaccinated four hours ago in perfect health, and now they're unresponsive, or seizing, with 105° fever, and labs, spinal tap, and imaging. I remind them that the child was vaccinated just hours before, but their notes say "encephalitis of unknown origin." I ask them if they'll file a VAERS report, and they say it's a coincidence. I remind them that VAERS is for reporting *any* symptoms that follow vaccination, whether causally linked or not; and they say they're not filing, because it has nothing to do with it. Nor do they bring it up to the parents. It's a big sweep-it-under-the-rug thing: any mention of vaccination is removed or withheld from the record. It happens every day.[8]

THE VICP PROCESS

With the VAERS system as background, it should come as no surprise that damage claims submitted to the VICP stand far less chance of winning an award than of simply being certified as vaccine-related in the VAERS database.

As we saw, both the VAERS and the Vaccine Injury Compensation Program—the VICP or "Vaccine Court"—were created by the National Childhood Vaccine Injury Act of 1986. In Mary Holland's well-documented history, the law was designed with four main purposes in mind:

1. to create the infrastructure for a national immunization program;
2. to insulate the industry and the medical profession from liability;
3. to establish a program to compensate the injured; and
4. to promote safer vaccines.[9]

Within that broad framework, the VAERS system could be understood as a research tool for achieving the Act's long-range objectives, namely, numbers 1 and 4, and the VICP program as a mechanism for achieving its more immediate goals, that is, numbers 2 and 3. But although at first the VAERS database gave abundant lip service as an open-ended invitation to the general public to report every adverse reaction, no matter how rare or as yet unsubstantiated as vaccine-linked, its arbitrary exclusion of SIDS, autism, chronic, autoimmune diseases, and indeed every other adverse reaction not yet admitted onto its minimal and ever-shrinking list of "reportable events" left little doubt that the list was essentially a rehash of the industry's flawed "safety" studies, and that its overriding purpose was simply to keep both the number of admissible VICP claims and the size of eventual awards as small as possible.

How the VICP process is structured in theory, and how it functions in practice, are admirably summarized by Professor Holland and her colleagues:

> All the injuries on the Vaccine Injury Table were to have occurred within 30 days of vaccination, most within hours or a few days. If petitioners met the exact requirements of the specified injuries, they would not be required to litigate and would receive compensation through an administrative "no-fault" process. For injuries not listed, they would have to prove them, based on a preponderance of the evidence, a "more likely than not" standard.
>
> The VICP insulates manufacturers and healthcare practitioners from liability and requires that petitions be brought solely against HHS, the rationale

> being to insure a stable vaccine supply and to keep prices affordable. Compensation is paid out of a Vaccine Injury Trust Fund collected from an excise tax of $0.75 imposed on the sale of every vaccine.
>
> Petitioners try their cases before one of eight Special Masters of the Court of Federal Claims, who are the sole finders of fact and law. Congress intended the VICP to be informal, without reliance on the Federal rules of evidence and civil procedure, to be simpler and less costly for the petitioner.
>
> Petitioners may receive $250,000 in the event of a vaccine-related death and a maximum of $250,000 for pain and suffering; these caps have not changed since 1986; the Law also provides attorney's fees and costs. It requires that petitions be filed within 36 months of the first manifestation or significant aggravation of such injury, a limitation shorter than in many state statutes; it does not provide for plaintiffs who did not or could not discover their injury within that time period.
>
> The Law also restricts private liability in any court unless the petitioner files first in the VICP. Since 1988, no manufacturer was liable for vaccine-related injury or death "if it resulted from side effects that were unavoidable, in spite of the vaccination having been properly prepared and accompanied by proper directions and warnings." This wording also became the basis for the U.S. Supreme Court's decision in *Bruesewitz v. Wyeth*, 2011, that manufacturers are shielded from all liability, as well as from having to give accurate or complete information to anyone but doctors, who are responsible for providing CDC Vaccine Information Statements to recipients.
>
> The Federal Circuit Court of Appeals has established that a petitioner's burden of proof consists in having to establish 1) a medical theory causally connecting the vaccination and the injury; 2) a logical sequence of cause and effect showing that the vaccine was the reason for the injury; and 3) a proximate temporal relationship between the vaccination and the injury. They are not required to show the precise mechanism, but merely that the vaccine in question caused the injury.[10]

As we saw with the VAERS system, the original rationale and official wording of the statute, the informality of the procedure, and the lower burden of proof all give the impression of benefiting the plaintiff; but its practical effect is quite the opposite. Once again, in the words of Professor Holland and her colleague,

> In the name of protecting children's health, the Act changed the legal landscape fundamentally. Instead of keeping doctors and the vaccine industry directly

> liable for adverse reactions to vaccines, it created a taxpayer-financed compensation program, in effect, a corporate bailout for the pharmaceutical injury, forcing the public to pay for "unavoidably unsafe" products, and thus depriving children of their most significant legal protections to insure safety and remedial compensation: informed consent and the right to sue manufacturers directly.
>
> So far, as of 2011, the HHS has compensated about 2,500 claims of vaccine-related death or injury with over $2 billion, including legal fees. The idea is simply that if children are injured, society has an ethical duty to care for them, just as for soldiers injured while serving in the military. Congress gave bipartisan support, and intended compensation to be quick, easy, certain, and generous.
>
> The reality has not lived up to the principle. The government goes to great lengths to compensate as few cases as possible, maintaining the fallacy that injuries are vanishingly rare. The VICP is a dismal failure. Almost 4 out of 5 claimants lose; the tenor of the proceedings is hostile and adversarial; almost no injuries are settled administratively, based on the Table; and cases take many years to litigate. It is referred to as a court, but it isn't a court: there is no judge, no jury, no right to require the adversary to provide information, and no formal rules of evidence and civil procedure.[11]

In 1999, Dr. David Satcher, then Surgeon-General of the United States, testified before Congress that VAERS receives about 11,000 to 12,000 reports of possible adverse vaccine reactions every year.[12] Given the admittedly vast extent of underreporting, this figure could represent anywhere from 10% of the actual number, as the CDC claims, to 1%, as in the FDA's estimate, or to 0.1%, as the ER nurse estimated from her years of service in "the trenches," which adds up to an average of 115,000, 1,150,000, or 11,500,000 children annually who suffer an adverse reaction that their parents sincerely believe to have been caused by a vaccine or vaccines: an enormous range, to be sure, but certainly more than enough in any case to give the lie to the usual assertion that these agents are overwhelmingly safe, unless you persist in the belief that most of these parents are either lying or stupid, and that what happened to their children was either a coincidence or never happened at all.

As one would expect, the number of VICP claims filed is much smaller, since payment is awarded only when vaccination is shown to have caused the injury more probably than not, and death or permanent disability has resulted. As of July 1, 2015, the official VICP website lists the following statistics regarding all claims filed since the beginning of the program, October 1, 1988:[13]

Total VICP claims filed: 16,038
- Death: 1,164
- Injury: 14,874

Claims compensated: 4,150
- By concession: 203
- By court decision: 172
- By settlement: 1,530

Claims dismissed: 9,912
Claims pending: 1,976

Over that same period, the 4,150 awards totaled approximately $3.18 billion. According to the website, over 80% of them represented "a negotiated settlement between the parties, in which HHS has not concluded, based upon review of the evidence, that the alleged vaccines caused the alleged injury." The stated reasons for settling include (1) a mutual decision "to minimize the risk of loss," (2) "a desire to minimize the time and expense of litigating," and (3) "the need to resolve a case quickly."[14]

At first glance, the fact that less than 5% of the awards were adjudicated in a formal hearing could be taken to mean that the government is generous enough to pay even when denying any vaccine link; but that impression is belied by the fact that over 95% of the awards *were* contested by the government and that only 6.4% of the total number of claims filed were found to be credible, based on the guidelines set forth in the VAERS system and the VICP Vaccine Injury Table.

If they were serious about insuring that compensation be "quick, easy, certain, and generous," that dismal track record would be reason enough to change the guidelines. Under these circumstances, it is easy to understand why petitioners feel they have little choice but to accept whatever the government offers, since their likelihood of success in a formal proceeding is almost nil, and indeed incalculable, since most people end up settling anyway.

About the closest we can come is to divide the number of claims compensated through adjudication (203) by the total number of claims heard in court without being conceded or settled (i.e., the number dismissed—9,912—plus the 203 successfully adjudicated, for a total of 10,115); 203 divided by 10,115 yields a probability of almost exactly 2% of prevailing in the Vaccine Court for those plaintiffs who refuse to settle and insist on taking their claims that far. So much for generosity. For the same money, and even with the same strict guidelines, they could have helped a lot more victims by simply avoiding the formal, court-like proceedings, which would save them not only the plaintiffs' legal and physician-witness fees, but also the salary of the Special Master and the fees of their own physician-witnesses.

With many claimants already assuming the enormous financial burden of their children's medical expenses, a major additional pressure on them to settle is the delay involved in formal proceedings, which in the cases I have written reports for amounted to a minimum of 2 years, and in death cases an average of 5–7 years, while more than a few last a decade or more, according to Wayne Rohde, author of *The Vaccine Court*, the most complete and up-to-date account of the program.[15]

SOME VICP CASES OF MY OWN

In 2002, I was engaged by a local attorney to review the medical records and write formal reports in support of the VICP claims of several adults and adolescents who had developed ongoing illnesses that they attributed to the hepatitis B vaccine. I can't say that they are representative of the program as a whole, (1) because the VICP was originally developed for infants and children, whereas the patients whose records I reviewed were two adolescent girls, one young adult, and three mature adults, (2) because they all revolved around just one vaccine, the Hep B, and (3) because I never met or spoke to any of them personally.

But since the hours of study required to prepare and file reports about them were enough for me to get to know them as well as some of my own patients, I decided to present the relevant details here, simply to provide some real-life accounts of how the VICP program actually functions. While differing from one another in their pathological diagnoses and the organs and tissues involved, they all shared some type of underlying autoimmune pathology, as I've come to expect in my other Hep B cases, and indeed in most if not all of the other vaccines as well.

Clinical reasoning and individualization should be the *sine qua non* for adjudicating VICP claims, because they arise from a singular misfortune that has already occurred, so that the hearing officer has no other duty beyond deciding whether, and to what extent, the particular illness or injury was caused or precipitated by a vaccine or vaccines and is therefore compensable under Federal law. But these quasi-judicial proceedings are consistently marred by dogmatic reliance on the same rigid guidelines and flawed assumptions that made a mockery of both the safety trials and the VAERS reports in the first place.

I have already cited the case of a young lab technician who became ill after her first round of Hep B shots. She showed no antibodies to the virus four years later, was mistakenly assumed to be still susceptible, and was therefore given a second round, as a result of which she developed autoimmune thyroiditis and an impressive array of other chronic complaints soon afterward. Very predictably, her case was dismissed without a hearing, according to the official guidelines, although purely on clinical grounds it was the most clear-cut of any in my experience.[16]

Here was a healthy young woman who from the chronology alone was clearly and seriously damaged by the vaccine, and should have received a sizable award. But because neither thyroiditis nor any of her other ailments were listed on the official Vaccine Injury Table, she was required to prove the legitimacy of her claim in an expensive and time-consuming process, yet she never even received a formal hearing. Following the VICP's imposed burden of proof, as outlined above, I submitted the following arguments:

> *As to plausibility,* the adverse reactions I have seen from hepatitis B vaccine are always of the autoimmune type. I added a case report of my own.
>
> *As to the medical literature,* I cited a large number of case reports of diverse autoimmune disorders traced to the Hep B vaccine, including systemic lupus and rheumatoid arthritis.
>
> *As to her illness,* I provided the history as above, and her own summary: "For the first 28 years of my life, I lived without being hospitalized other than for giving birth to my son. Other than hay-fever symptoms in spring and fall, I rarely got sick or went to the doctor. But things changed drastically after those shots."
>
> *As to the chronology,* her illness began within a few days after the first dose of the vaccine, and intensified after each additional dose, too soon for any other causal factor to merit serious consideration.
>
> *As to any other possible causes,* there were none. There was nothing in her history, other than the prolonged illness after her first round of hepatitis B vaccine, which gave fair warning not to repeat it.[17]

Another four years passed before the VICP arbitrarily disposed of her claim without a hearing, based on the official guidelines.

My second case was that of a thirteen-year-old girl who was already ill with type 1 diabetes, but had been in stable condition for several years, until soon after her first dose of Hep B vaccine, when she developed a number of crippling allergies she had never had before:

> An adolescent girl with insulin-dependent juvenile diabetes was in stable condition and otherwise in good health before receiving the vaccine. Within a few days of her first dose, she developed fatigue and malaise, her skin became swollen and puffy, and she itched intensely from hives that appeared all over her body. In the ensuing weeks she also developed joint pains, and the hives, itching, and scratching all intensified to the point of drawing blood. Medications brought only temporary relief.
>
> Her elevated sedimentation rate and anti-nuclear antibody titer pointed to an autoimmune disease resembling systemic lupus, but vigorous treatment didn't help; and she soon developed allergic reactions to chemicals and food additives that had never bothered her before, while her diabetes, which had been stable for years, went seriously out of control.
>
> After several months, her mother broke off the treatment, saying, "Before the shot, she was active, full of life, not allergic to anything. Now she has to analyze whatever she eats, avoid the sun, and take her EpiPen wherever she goes. She is allergic to preservatives and food colorings, but has no idea what else will trigger hives and rashes."[18]

Her case was settled for $5,000 three years after it was filed. Perhaps the award was so meager because of her preexisting condition, which might have encouraged the government's physicians to make light of her allergies as part of its natural progression. But that is precisely why her case and others like it need to be thought about more carefully, since everyone, no matter how healthy, has latent tendencies to react to antigenic stimuli in various ways; and it would be obvious to any practicing physician that the vaccination exacerbated her preexisting condition and caused it to spread to other areas that had never been involved before. In both respects, it resembles many of my other non-VICP cases that I discussed previously, where the vaccines seemed to act mainly in this nonspecific way, to exacerbate the ear infections, asthma, and whatever other conditions were already present.

A further detail is that type 1 diabetes is itself an autoimmune disease that has been linked to several vaccines, leaving us free to wonder how she acquired it in the first place, since we are totally ignorant of her previous vaccine history, and evidently none of her pediatricians thought it relevant to mention it.

Here is a third case, which I present precisely because it was by far the most severe of them all, and also involved a long and complicated past history of peripheral vascular disease that was already serious enough to cast doubt on any causal link to the vaccine without paying close attention to the pertinent clinical details:

With a long history of intermittent claudication, a 55-year-old police officer suffered ischemic occlusion of his abdominal aorta at the age of 34 and underwent an aorto-femoral bypass graft and resection of his left popliteal artery, both of which proved very successful. Although his application for early retirement and disability was rejected, through determination, hard work, and a rigorous program of exercise and physical therapy he eventually returned to the force. Eleven years later, however, a femoral arteriogram revealed significant narrowing of the lower portion of the left femoral artery and aneurysmal dilatation above it, indicating a high risk of thrombosis and further complications in the future, all ample grounds for exempting him from the Hepatitis B vaccine requirement in the first place.

In spite of his misgivings, he was told that his health insurance would be cancelled if he refused; so he reluctantly agreed to take it. Within a few days after the first dose, he developed a flu-like illness, with fever, muscle aches, a skin rash, eye pain, and blurred vision, a picture closely resembling the "hypersensitivity syndrome" listed in the *PDR* as a side-effect of the vaccine. In spite of repeated assurances that the vaccine was harmless and couldn't possibly cause such a reaction, his symptoms persisted for weeks, making him even more hesitant about the second dose; but once again he had little choice but to accept the ruling of the Health Department that the vaccine was safe and required for his employment.

Within hours of receiving the second dose, he developed symptoms that were much more intense, chiefly earache, tinnitus, loss of vision, overpowering fatigue, asthma, and high blood pressure, as a result of which the third dose was postponed for 6 months. In spite of this long delay, his reaction to it was the most violent of all. Within a few days, he developed severe tinnitus, hearing loss, inability to urinate, and an intensely dark-purple, petechial rash; his diagnosis was "malignant hypertension." A week later, his blood pressure had remained dangerously high, even after strong medication.

Over the next few months, he experienced frequent headaches, dizziness, visual field defects, and attacks of unilateral blindness lasting up to 30 minutes, as a result of which he consulted an ophthalmologist and was diagnosed with "ophthalmic migraine," but the medications given for it were ineffective. After 40 or 50 such episodes made it impossible for him to perform his duties, he was finally granted a disability pension; but within a few weeks he was hospitalized for chest pain, malaise, and low urine output, at which time his blood pressure, cholesterol, triglycerides, BUN, and creatinine were all found to be dangerously high, and he was given the diagnosis of acute renal failure.

> Finding specific antibodies to various fatty substances in the blood, his physician finally made the additional diagnosis of "anti-phospholipid syndrome," an autoimmune disorder that poses serious risks of death from thrombosis anywhere in the body, and finally connected the dots of his various ailments to the Hepatitis B vaccine as a result of similar case reports in the literature. Over the past 8 years since that episode, his symptoms have persisted in spite of aggressive treatment, along with severe hypertension and chronic renal impairment. Now permanently disabled, he remains at high risk, not only for stroke and heart attack, but also for further progression of his peripheral vascular disease, (i.e., gangrene of the lower extremities), as well as blindness and end-stage kidney failure, with very poor chances of living out a normal life span.[19]

Nevertheless, his VICP claim was dismissed without a hearing. Although I don't know the exact reasons, the life-threatening antiphospholipid syndrome is not listed on the Vaccine Injury Table, and his peripheral vascular disease was already far advanced, and had continued to worsen long before he was vaccinated. Since autoimmune phenomena were still off-limits in any event, I surmise that the government doctors simply wrote it off as an exacerbation of his pre-existing condition. But that is precisely why I wanted to present his case; as before, the clinical perspective of the practicing physician removes any doubt as to the causal role of the vaccine, even granting his extensive past history.

Once again, it seems fitting to conclude this chapter with the words of Barbara Loe Fisher, who helped write the National Childhood Vaccine Injury Act of 1986. She has devoted the past thirty-five years of her life to organizing for safer vaccines and advocating for vaccine-injured children and their parents. Perhaps better than anyone else, she knows the entire, sad history of the VAERS reporting system and the VICP program, which her principled activism did so much to create, and now feels obliged to call it out for what it has become:

> In 1982, as parent of a DPT-injured child, I was invited to testify before Congress after the drug companies threatened to stop distributing childhood vaccines unless they were shielded from liability. We fought to protect the right to sue them for injuries and deaths under the National Childhood Vaccine Injury Act. Both politicians and the American Academy of Pediatrics and politicians called the VICP program "simple justice" and "a safety net" for children.
>
> When Congress gave partial liability protection to the industry and the doctors, we were promised that the VICP program would be quick, easy, non-adversarial, and less traumatic and expensive than a lawsuit, without

prohibiting such lawsuits. We trusted Congress to keep its promises to inform parents and improve vaccine safety, by requiring drug companies to conduct research, Federal health agencies to identify high-risk children, and pediatricians to report adverse reactions to the VAERS system.

Every one of these promises has been broken. Over the past 30 years, government agencies, drug companies, and doctors have turned the VICP program into a parent's worst nightmare. Congress and the Supreme Court have declared that vaccines are "unavoidably unsafe" and banned lawsuits against the industry, while government officials insist that vaccines are 100% safe, so that it's our fault when something bad happens.

Even if genetic, biological, and environmental differences increase our susceptibility to vaccine reactions, the law creating the VICP affirms that children with pre-existing conditions made worse after vaccination are still entitled to compensation. In 2014, a GAO report affirmed what parents have said for years, that CDC officials have dropped several adverse reactions from the Vaccine Injury Table for the sole purpose of denying compensation to vaccine-injured children.

In this and so many other ways, the VICP program has betrayed the public trust:

1. By 2015, over $3 billion has been awarded to more than 4,000 child and adult vaccine victims; but 2 out of 3 children applying for compensation are turned down, despite a $3-billion surplus in the Vaccine Injury Trust Fund.
2. In the early years of the program, most vaccine-injured children were compensated without a hearing. But in 1995, the CDC changed the rules, and the system became highly adversarial. Today, very few vaccine-injured children qualify for an uncontested award, especially in cases of permanent brain damage
3. Today, 80% of awards are given to adults disabled by flu shots, which are optional, and only 20% to children required to get vaccinated to attend daycare or school.
4. Most claims take years to adjudicate, because HHS and the DOJ spend tax dollars to deny compensation to the majority of children and adults who apply for it.
5. Parents are not told about the 2- to 3-year deadlines for filing a claim, and so regularly miss them.
6. Many pediatricians refuse to comply with the informing, recording and reporting provisions for vaccine safety in the law, and some even refuse to care for children whose parents don't comply with the CDC vaccine schedule.

> In short, the VICP program is a failed experiment. Years of neglect and failure to provide oversight have allowed both government and industry to undermine the program to the point that it cannot and should not be salvaged. It is time to repeal the 1986 law and again hold drug companies accountable for the risks and failures of vaccination in a court of law.[20]

SUMMARY

The "Vaccine Court" originated as a well-intentioned response to popular agitation for fast, easy, and generous compensation of the growing number of vaccine injuries and deaths; but as so often happens in an ostensibly democratic republic favoring the rich and powerful, it was hijacked by the industry to shield them from liability. The result has been the caricature of a real court, with no judge, no jury, and no clear rules of evidence or legal procedure,

- in which claimants receive a disposition based on arbitrary and unrealistic criteria;
- in which the probability of success is vanishingly small;
- in which a minimum of several years are consumed in the process; and
- in which the fundamental legal right of seeking redress against the manufacturer has been taken away.

In retrospect, they would be considerably better off taking their chances in a court of law, as they did before the VICP was created.

PART III

THE RESEARCH PERSPECTIVE

Chapter 9

EPIDEMIOLOGY AND CLINICAL RESEARCH

As we saw, most universities, hospitals, and medical schools can no longer afford to fund large-scale, prospective clinical trials, and have turned to the vaccine manufacturers for financial support. What they have given up in exchange is control over the design, the conduct, and even the results of their experiments, and thus ultimately their cherished commitment to scientific objectivity. Lacking comparable resources of their own, independent investigators have had to rely for the most part on population surveys involving questionnaires and incidence figures, and retrospective clinical studies of medical records regarding adverse events that have already taken place.

In this chapter, I have reviewed both types of evidence together, because they are essentially complementary. While not rising quite to the level of conclusive proof, they nevertheless provide highly suggestive evidence for the adverse effects of vaccination that is difficult to ignore.

THE INFANT MORTALITY RATE

Widely accepted as one of the most accurate indicators of a country's general level of health, the infant mortality rate (IMR) measures the rate of infant deaths in the first year of life per 100,000 live births. For decades now, epidemiologists have puzzled over the apparent paradox that the United States, which ranks near the top of all countries in the level of sanitation and the extent of its public health infrastructure, has nevertheless consistently maintained by far the highest IMR in the developed world, currently, 6.2 per 100,000, as compared with less than 2.8 per 100,000 in Japan and Sweden at the low end.

In 2011, suspecting a link with our aggressive vaccination policy, Miller and Goldman studied the United States and the 33 countries with IMRs lower than ours in relation to the total vaccine load administered to infants in the first year of life, not counting Third World nations whose minimal levels of sanitation and public health infrastructure guarantee IMRs much higher than any of those listed. Further excluding Andorra, Liechtenstein, San Marino, and Monaco, tiny states with less than 5 deaths each, they subdivided the 30 remaining countries into 5 groups, according to the total number of vaccine doses mandated in the first year, based on the 2008–2009 schedules, and counting each component of the MMR, DTaP, and other vaccine combinations as separate doses:

Group 1. 12–14 doses:
Sweden, Japan, Iceland, Norway, Denmark, Finland

Group 2. 15–17 doses:
Malta, Slovenia, South Korea, Singapore, New Zealand

Group 3. 18–20 doses:
Germany, Switzerland, Israel, Italy, France, Czech Republic, Belgium, UK, Spain

Group 4. 21–23 doses:
Portugal, Luxembourg, Cuba, Austria, Ireland, Greece

Group 5. 24–26 doses:
Netherlands, Canada, Australia, US[1]

Just as they had suspected, the authors found that the average IMR of each group was directly proportional to the total number of required vaccine doses that defined it:

Group	Average Doses	Average IMR[2]
1	13	3.36
2	16	3.89
3	19	4.28
4	22	4.97
5	25	5.19

Once again, the United States easily topped both lists, with by far the highest IMR of all nations included in the analysis, and the most required vaccinations in the first year, amounting to 26 doses in 2011, more than any other country in the world. In short, the evidence seems clear enough

1. that nations requiring the most vaccine doses in the first year show the highest infant mortality rates, and
2. that those requiring the fewest doses, mainly the Scandinavian countries and Japan, are the healthiest in that fundamental sense.[3]

Multiple Vaccines as a Cause of Death and Poor General Health

Another study by the same authors considered the effect on mortality and the rate of hospitalization from giving multiple vaccines and vaccine components simultaneously, addressing an early concern voiced by Dr. Wakefield regarding the triple MMR vaccine, and echoing a number of anecdotal reports of infants dying soon after receiving a hexavalent vaccine, for example, or similar "cocktails" of several different vaccines at once. Analyzing the raw data of nearly 39,000 adverse reactions reported to the VAERS system between 1990 and 2010, and again counting each component of multiple vaccines like the MMR or DTaP as separate doses, they found

1. that infants receiving 6, 7, or 8 vaccine doses simultaneously were significantly more likely to be hospitalized afterwards than those receiving 2, 3, or 4 doses, and
2. that infants receiving 5–8 vaccine doses simultaneously were significantly more likely to die afterwards than those receiving 1–4 doses.[4]

In a third study by a different author, children receiving all vaccines on the official CDC-recommended schedule were compared with those who received a smaller number. Analyzing the health records of nearly 325,000 American children under two years of age who were enrolled in eight managed-care organizations, the authors found that the "under-vaccinated" children were significantly less likely to require outpatient visits, ER visits, and hospitalizations than those who were up-to-date: "Children under-vaccinated because of parental choice had significantly lower utilization rates of both Emergency Department and outpatient settings, both overall and for specific acute illnesses, than children who were vaccinated on schedule."[5]

Moreover, children who were vaccinated the least showed the greatest reductions; and the differences might have been greater still had the study included ER and inpatient visits in the first 8 days of life, at least some of which could have been linked to the mandate that the hepatitis B vaccine be given at birth.

All three studies provide overlapping, mutually reinforcing evidence of a linear or proportional relationship between infant morbidity and mortality, on the one hand, and the total number of vaccine doses administered early in life on the other. What particularly stood out about these findings is

1. that they redirect attention to the generic, nonspecific effects of the vaccination process itself, rather than the specific effects of any particular vaccine;
2. that they validate the instinctive fear, articulated by so many parents but routinely dismissed by their doctors, that the total number of vaccines administered is indeed important, and that far too many are being given; and
3. that the generic, nonspecific effect of multiple vaccinations helps explain why the vast bulk of adverse reactions to vaccines are so easily missed, and so rarely looked for.

WHERE ARE THE UNVACCINATED?

On the other hand, even the "under-vaccinated" children just cited and those living in countries with the fewest mandates still receive a significant number of shots. In societies such as ours, where many vaccines are multiple to begin with, and often combined with others at a typical well-baby visit, clearly the most accurate way to evaluate the broad effect of vaccination on large populations would be to compare two groups of children, matched demographically as closely as possible, one fully vaccinated according to the official CDC schedule, and the other not vaccinated at all. It boggles the mind that our country, which yields to none in its professed commitment to science, has never undertaken such a simple and practical survey, or even proposed it as a good idea.

A further consequence is that the kids whose parents choose not to vaccinate them, although still comprising but a tiny fraction of all children in America, are the indispensable control group for investigating the true impact of the vaccination process in the unbiased, objective manner that real science requires, and thus deserve our gratitude and admiration, rather than the bullying and opprobrium they typically receive, in making valid research possible in a society where so many vaccinations are required of everyone else.

The Amish

One such population that hasn't yet received the attention it deserves are the Amish, most of whom still live in a simple, old-fashioned way, grow their own organic food, and don't vaccinate their children. In 2009, Dan Olmsted, a United Press International reporter, set out to investigate the legendary belief that Amish children seldom, if ever, develop autism, and was surprised to learn that the CDC wasn't interested in finding out why, or even whether it was true:

> The rate of autism among the Amish is so low that if it were the same in the rest of the population, we wouldn't even be talking about it. In 2005 I wrote, "Where are the autistic Amish? Here in Pennsylvania Dutch country, there should be well over 100 with some form of it. I've come here to find them, but so far have failed."
>
> In northeastern Ohio, the nation's largest Amish community, Dr. Wiznitzer, a CDC spokesperson, said the incidence was 1 in 10,000. So in the US, with an autism rate of 66 per 10,000, that's one sixty-sixth of the going rate! Why is the rate so much lower, and why doesn't anyone in authority seem to care?
>
> In June 2005, the autism rate for US children was 1 in 166, according to the CDC, while for the Amish around Middlefield, Ohio, Dr. Heng Wang, Medical Director of the Clinic that treats them, is aware of just one 12-year-old boy with autism, out of the 15,000 Amish children living there. He says that half of them were vaccinated, including the autistic boy, by the way, and half weren't. But, vaccinated or not, 1 in 15,000 is a very low rate![6]

Finally, in 2014, several years after UPI discontinued his series, Sharyl Attkisson, the intrepid CBS reporter whom we've met before, latched on to the story, contacted a CDC official for comment and posted an article about their conversation:

> I told her that a survey of this unvaccinated population could be a first step in dispelling or confirming the possibility of a vaccine tie to autism. It wouldn't cost much, because the CDC already conducts surveys to monitor vaccination coverage; it need only add whether or not each child has been diagnosed with Autism Spectrum. If the incidence of autism is roughly the same in kids regard-

less of vaccinations, it would help those wanting to debunk a vaccine-autism link. But if the incidence is markedly lower or higher in the unvaccinated, it would be grounds for serious study.

She reluctantly agreed that somebody should do it. "Why not the CDC?" I asked. Dr. Bernardine Healy, former head of the NIH, suggested that Federal officials don't want to do such studies because they're afraid of the evidence of a vaccine-autism link, and how it would impact vaccination rates globally.[7]

VACCINATED AND UNVACCINATED IN NEW ZEALAND

In 1992, the Immunisation Awareness Society of New Zealand conducted a survey of vaccinated and unvaccinated children in that country; participants were asked about common childhood ailments, such as asthma, eczema, tonsillitis, ear infections, hyperactivity, diabetes, and epilepsy, as well as developmental delays in sitting up, crawling, and walking.

Questionnaires were distributed informally through IAS members, friends, and associates; of the 245 families who responded, by no means all were IAS members, and their 495 children included 226 who were vaccinated and 269 who were not. What "vaccinated" actually meant (i.e., exactly *how many* vaccinations each child received) was not reported; and several families included older children who were vaccinated fully or partially, and younger ones who were not, a result paralleling my own experience that parents who take the trouble to educate themselves often stop vaccinating the children they already have, as well as those yet to be born in the future.

Among the respondents, both members and nonmembers were also significantly more likely to breast-feed their children than mothers in the general population, and be more health-conscious in other respects as well. But to the extent that any or all of these issues mattered, they would have tended to blur the differences between the groups, which were very similar demographically and thus extremely well matched in other respects as well, a homogeneity that makes the wide discrepancies that were actually observed even more striking:[8]

	Vaccinated (n=226)	% of total	Unvaccinated (n=269)	% of total
Asthma	34	15.04	8	2.97
Eczema	63	27.88	34	12.64
Recurrent otitis	56	24.78	16	5.95
Tonsillitis	26	11.50	3	1.12
Tonsillectomy	12	5.31	0	0.00
Apnea	14	6.19	4	1.49
Hyperactivity	13	5.75	4	1.49
Epilepsy	4	1.77	0	0.00

In summary, the author emphasized the remarkable uniformity and lack of ambiguity in these results, even allowing for the smallness of the sample:

> The results overwhelmingly show that unvaccinated children suffer far less from chronic childhood conditions than those vaccinated, with significant differences in asthma, eczema, ear infections, and tonsillitis. While this was a very limited study in the numbers of unvaccinated children involved and the range of chronic conditions investigated, it provides solid scientific evidence that unvaccinated children are significantly healthier than their vaccinated peers.[9]

It should also be kept in mind that this survey was published in 1992 when many fewer vaccines were required, so that the resulting differences would almost certainly be even greater if comparable populations were studied today, as they clearly should be.

To summarize, I take it as further corroboration of these surveys, as of what has been said in earlier chapters, that their results all point in the same direction:

1. that vaccinations adversely affect the general health of populations receiving them;
2. that they do so in more or less direct proportion to the total number of vaccines given; and
3. that most of the harm they cause is therefore inherent in the nature of the vaccination process, and not merely the specific effect of this or that particular vaccine.

ALLERGIES AND ASTHMA

Some pro-vaccine advocates have challenged these results, contending not implausibly that the parents of unvaccinated children generally prefer more natural approaches, and are less likely to trust physicians and hospitals or seek their care, so the illnesses of their children are less likely to be reported or diagnosed. Since that argument would carry less weight in the case of serious and potentially life-threatening or disabling illnesses, which very few parents are prepared to treat on their own without trained medical supervision, I decided to focus more narrowly on adverse reactions that qualify as major diseases.

In a 1994 study of 446 children averaging 8 years of age who had nursed for more than a year and received only breast milk for the first six months, the 243 who were vaccinated against pertussis were compared with the 203 who were not, with the result that 26 of the vaccinated group, or 10.7%, later developed asthma, while only 4, or 2%, of the unvaccinated controls did so.[10] Another study of 1,265 children born in Christchurch, New Zealand, found that 23% of those receiving the DTP and polio vaccines developed episodes of asthma before the age of ten, 22.5% consulted specialists for it, and 30% consulted specialists for other types of allergies, whereas none of the children who were not vaccinated suffered any such episodes, or required any such consultations; similar discrepancies were observed at 5 and 16 years of age.[11]

SEIZURES

Similarly, a number of research teams have documented a significantly higher risk of seizures following a variety of different vaccines, including the DTaP, polio (IPV), Hib, pneumococcus, and MMR. One Danish study analyzed a population of 378,834 children who received the DTaP, IPV, and Hib vaccines simultaneously on 3 separate occasions, as recommended by the CDC, and found that they were 8 times more likely to have febrile seizures on the day of the first series, and 4 times more likely to have them on the day of the second series, than at other times.[12] In addition, those adding the pneumococcus vaccine to each cocktail had a still higher risk of seizures on the day of each series, and for three days following the second series.[13]

Nevertheless, the authors were at pains to reassure their readers that these febrile seizures did *not* lead to chronic epilepsy:

> Within seven years of follow-up, 2,248 children were diagnosed with epilepsy, 131 of them unvaccinated and 2117 vaccinated. Among the 2,117 who received the shot, 813 were diagnosed between 3 and 15 months and 1,304 were diagnosed later in life; but only two children were diagnosed with epilepsy on the day of the first vaccination and only one on the day of the second. Compared with the unvaccinated cohort, the vaccinated children had a lower risk of epilepsy in the first 15 months of life, but [had] a similar risk of epilepsy afterward.[14]

Unfortunately, this conclusion was based on a well-crafted deception. In fact, *there were no unvaccinated children,* as was explained in the fine print:

> Vaccination was treated as a time-dependent variable. Children entered the reference cohort at the beginning of follow-up and moved to the exposed cohort on the day of vaccination. The children remained in the exposed cohort for eight days and then returned to the reference cohort until the day of the next vaccination.[15]

In other words, *all* of the children were vaccinated; they were put into the unvaccinated or "reference" group until the day of their vaccinations, when they were moved into the vaccinated or "exposed" group, kept there for only 8 days, and then moved back to the unvaccinated group. So all that was being compared was the risk of developing epilepsy in the 8 days immediately following each series, and the risk of the same children developing epilepsy at any other time—as if an adverse reaction occurring outside that narrow window were somehow not vaccine-related.

This strategy is obviously another version of that commonly employed in the manufacturers' safety trials, as detailed in the package inserts and described in chapter 3; and in this case, it would have been entirely acceptable, had the authors not misnamed the control group "unvaccinated," to lull the reader into believing that it consisted of different children rather than the very same ones, and thus gloss over the well-known tendency for febrile seizures to progress at times to full-blown epilepsy, and for adverse reactions to vaccines to include it and other chronic diseases that often require weeks, months, or even years to develop.

In fact, just such a progression was clearly documented in a retrospective study of 247 cases of vaccine-related seizures taken from the German national database between 2006 and 2008, which showed that 49% were febrile, while

12.6% represented ongoing, non-febrile epileptic syndromes, and 8.5% were described as *status epilepticus,* a life-threatening emergency.[16]

TYPE 1 DIABETES

In like manner, a number of studies have shown that children receiving the pertussis, Hib, MMR, and hepatitis B vaccines run significantly higher risks of developing type 1 or insulin-dependent diabetes mellitus (IDDM), yet another autoimmune disease, than unvaccinated children. In one retrospective study, for example, 240,000 children were divided into three groups, based on whether they had received no doses, one dose, or four doses of the Hib vaccine as infants; the incidence of type 1 diabetes was then calculated for each group, at both 7 and 10 years of age. At ages 7 and 10, there were, respectively, 26% and 33.4% more cases of type 1 diabetes in the group receiving four doses than in the unvaccinated group.[17] In addition, the authors found that most extra cases developed at 36–48 months after the shots, a significant clustering that supported a causal relationship,[18] while mice receiving the Hib vaccine likewise showed a higher risk of developing the disease.[19] The same authors also discovered a comparable time lag of 2 to 4 years between MMR vaccination and a definite clustering of type 1 diabetes cases, as well as a comparable decline in the disease when the BCG vaccine was discontinued.[20]

Turning his attention to the Hep B vaccine, the lead author subsequently found that children given the Hep B vaccine in New Zealand, Italy, and France were also at significantly higher risk for developing type 1 diabetes than those who did not receive it.[21] In New Zealand, for example, the incidence of IDDM rose by 48% in children up to 14 years of age after the Hep B vaccination was mandated,[22] while in France the incidence of IDDM in children up to 4 years old increased by 60% after Hep B vaccination was introduced, and showed a second spike at 10–14 years of age.[23]

Other significant findings were the clustering of cases developing 2 to 4 years after the series, once again supporting a causal link,[24] and a major time lag between the vaccination and the appearance of the disease, years in this instance, whereas any adverse reaction occurring more than a few days after a vaccination had previously been a standard basis for writing it off, and thus for automatically ruling out chronic diseases more or less by definition.

Such consistent findings for so many different vaccines have led the same author to hypothesize that *all* vaccines are capable of inducing IDDM in susceptible children, such as those with a positive family history of the disease, particularly in a sibling.[25] His statistical analysis of 11 years of health data showed

1. that Hib, MMR, OPV, and DTaP were all associated with a higher risk of type 1 diabetes;[26]
2. that a single dose of MMR increased the risk by 88%, and that two doses of OPV doubled the risk;[27] and
3. that a child with a sibling with the disease is 70–150 times more likely to develop IDDM from a Hib vaccine than to derive any benefit from it.[28]

HEMORRHAGIC DISEASES

A growing number of vaccines, namely, the MMR, pertussis, chicken pox, influenza, and hepatitis A and B, have also been causally linked to idiopathic thrombocytopenic purpura (ITP), a potentially life-threatening, autoimmune bleeding disorder, characterized by a low platelet count and external and/or internal bleeding at multiple sites. Inasmuch as hemorrhagic phenomena have long been recognized as a complication of measles and rubella infections, MMR was an obvious suspect. A 2014 article found that ITP is five times more likely to occur after MMR,[29] while an Italian study found a comparably increased risk for a period of six weeks afterward.[30]

But just as with IDDM, similar associations have been documented for a number of other vaccines as well. In 2016, for example, hematologists at an Osaka hospital reported three cases of ITP in elderly Japanese patients:[31]

1. a woman of 81, hospitalized with ITP four weeks after receiving a flu vaccine, with a low platelet count of 39,000;
2. a woman of 75, hospitalized for oral and nasal hemorrhaging five weeks after her flu shot, with a platelet count of only 5,000; and
3. a woman of 87, hospitalized for vaginal bleeding and purpura just two weeks after a flu shot, with a platelet count of 2,000.

All three had been well prior to their vaccinations, with normal platelet counts, and were later successfully treated and discharged without further complications.

Another research team analyzed the health records of 1.8 million children and adolescents to assess their risk of developing ITP after their vaccinations.

They compared the incidence of the disease for a period of 42 days after each shot with the times before and after that period. The following is what they found:

1. For the MMR, in children 12–19 months of age, ITP was five times more likely in the 42-day period after the vaccine than before or after it.[32]
2. For the chicken pox vaccine, in children 11–17 years old, ITP was 12 times more likely in the same period after the shot than earlier or later.[33]
3. For the Tdap, in children 11–17 years old, ITP was 20 times more likely in the same post-vaccine period than earlier or later,[34]
4. For the Hep A vaccine, in children of 7–17, ITP is 23 times more likely in the post-vaccine period than earlier or later.[35]

VACCINATING PREMATURE INFANTS

So pervasive and widely believed is the myth of vaccine safety that even intelligent, well-trained neonatologists rarely have second thoughts about vaccinating their most vulnerable patients (i.e., premature and low-birth-weight babies in the Newborn ICU), even though a number of studies have documented life-threatening complications, chiefly apnea, bradycardia, oxygen desaturation, and cyanosis in these babies promptly after being vaccinated.

In 2007, for example, M. Pourcyrous and colleagues at the University of Tennessee selected 239 premature infants who were still in the NICU and on track to be vaccinated at two or more months of age; they divided them into two groups, giving one a single vaccine (either DTaP, Hib, Pneumo, Hep B, or IPV), and giving the others all of them simultaneously. This is what they found:

1. Seventy percent of the infants receiving a single vaccine, and 85% of those receiving the multi-dose cocktail, showed abnormally high levels of C-reactive protein,[36] a sign of acute inflammatory or autoimmune responses, and widely used in newborns as a warning of major infection or cardiorespiratory complication.
2. Sixteen percent of all the infants suffered major or life-threatening cardiorespiratory events within 48 hours following their shots (i.e., apnea, bradycardia, oxygen desaturation, and/or cyanosis).[37]
3. Thirty-two percent of the infants who were multiply vaccinated did so.[38]

4. The infants receiving the cocktail were 4 times more likely to suffer complications than those receiving only one vaccine, and 16 times more likely to show warning levels of C-reactive protein.[39]

Here is the authors' summary of their findings: "Our study revealed that some vaccines were associated with adverse cardio-respiratory events and abnormal CRP values in premature infants in the NICU, even when administered alone, and the incidence of these events was even higher following the simultaneous administration of multiple vaccines."[40]

The propensity of vaccines to provoke apnea, bradycardia, cyanosis, oxygen desaturation, and other life-threatening complications in premature infants has been confirmed in many other studies as well. A team from the Neonatology Unit at Children's Hospital in Geneva, Switzerland, for example, discovered that 33 of 64 preemies of very low birth weight, or 51.5%, experienced an adverse cardiorespiratory event following their first DTaP shot, and that six of these, or 18%, suffered a recurrence after their second one.[41] In 2001, a group of British neonatologists published similar findings:

1. Seventeen of 45 premature infants given DTaP and Hib vaccines in the NICU suffered adverse reactions soon afterward, for a rate of 37.8%.[42]
2. Nine of the 45, or 20%, suffered major complications, including apnea, bradycardia, and low oxygen saturation.[43]
3. All 9 were among the 27 vaccinated on or before their 70th day of life, for a rate of 33%.[44]

SUMMARY

Population-based surveys have shown a linear, directly proportional relationship between the number of vaccinations administered in the first year of life and the infant mortality rate, as well as the rate of hospitalizations and emergency room visits during the same period. Other surveys have shown that children vaccinated according to the CDC schedule exhibit higher rates of asthma and other childhood diseases and generally have poorer health than those who were "undervaccinated," while those children who were never vaccinated at all seemed by far the healthiest in a number of typical parameters. All of these studies were especially noteworthy for singling out not any particular vaccine, but rather the total vaccine *load*, the number of vaccinations given, and thus something in the nature of the vaccination process itself.

In addition, retrospective analyses of clinical data (i.e., hospital and outpatient visits), have shown that vaccinated children are significantly more prone to develop a number of important complications, namely, asthma, seizures, epilepsy, IDDM or type 1 diabetes, and autoimmune ITP, than their unvaccinated counterparts, and that premature infants were much more likely to develop major cardiorespiratory complications, mainly apnea, bradycardia, oxygen desaturation, and cyanosis, within 48 hours after being vaccinated than otherwise, especially within the first 70 days of life. A majority of preemies vaccinated during that period also showed abnormal elevations of C-reactive protein, a warning sign or precursor of inflammation, whether from infection or autoimmune phenomena. The studies of autoimmune diabetes were especially important in documenting a time lag of three to four years between being vaccinated and developing the disease, exactly as Shoenfeld and his colleagues have emphasized.

Finally, these studies are a kind of mirror image of the research cited in chapter 1, which showed that coming down with and recovering from many of the acute childhood illnesses that we typically vaccinate against help to prevent many serious chronic diseases later in life.

Chapter 10

THE LABORATORY SCIENCES

Over and above the clinical and epidemiological data showing the propensity of vaccines to cause death and a broad array of chronic diseases in susceptible individuals, the fundamental mystery of how vaccines really act inside the human body, whether for good or ill, has never been fully elucidated, while major portions of what is known lie buried and unread in medical and scientific journals, or have been allowed to remain closely guarded "trade secrets" to a shockingly great extent. In this chapter, I will present an introduction to valid research in the laboratory sciences, chiefly immunology, biochemistry, and microbiology, in an effort to fill in some of the blanks, especially in three specific areas:

1. the autoimmune mechanisms of mercury and aluminum toxicity;
2. autoimmune mechanisms as the principal pathway for how all vaccines act on everyone; and
3. the as yet largely unknown toxicity of other vaccine ingredients (contaminants, tissue culture cell lines, culture media, preservatives, detergents, etc.).

THIMEROSAL AND ETHYLMERCURY

Thimerosal, an organomercury derivative originally patented in the 1930s as the germicide Merthiolate, is still widely used as a preservative in vaccines, despite its proven ability to cross the blood-brain barrier and the known multisystem toxicity of mercury and the various compounds containing it, especially on the brain and central nervous system.

That its neurotoxicity involves an autoimmune mechanism was demonstrated by the simple expedient of injecting both thimerosal alone and vaccines prepared with it into genetically pure strains of newborn mice, with the predictable result that the autoimmune-susceptible strains exhibited stunted growth, abnormal behavior, and histopathological changes in their brain tissue, whereas the autoimmune-resistant strains did not.[1] As to the exact mechanisms involved, another study of newborn mice found the following:

1. Thimerosal causes brain damage in proportion to its content of ethylmercury, which is even more harmful than the methylmercury found in contaminated fish.
2. It damages dendritic cells of the brain and spinal cord, major elements of the cellular immune system, mainly by causing inflammation.
3. It causes excessive secretion of inflammatory cytokines such as interleukin-6, which promote inflammation in brain tissue.
4. It is a potent antioxidant, inhibiting oxidative phosphorylation, the basic aerobic pathway of energy production in the body, which utilizes oxygen, the citric acid cycle, and the high-energy phosphate bonds of ATP, with calcium ions (Ca^{++}) as a cofactor.[2]

This last finding is particularly important, because the brain accounts for only 2% of the total body mass, but consumes fully 20% of its inhaled oxygen,[3] and is therefore exquisitely vulnerable to any interference with this most basic and indispensable pathway.

In 2012, a related study investigating the effect of thimerosal on the biochemistry of astrocytes, a major group of glial cells in brain tissue that protects the neurons and supports their function, confirmed that its antioxidant effect is centered in the mitochondria, the area of the cell where oxidative phosphorylation is mainly carried out, and involves overproduction of "reactive oxygen states," resulting in hyperpolarization and breakage of the mitochondrial membrane, loss of signal, and ultimately shrinkage and disintegration of the cell.[4]

As for the gross neuropathological changes found at autopsy, a team of Polish anatomists injected newborn rats with four doses of thimerosal, at 7, 9, 11, and 15 days, respectively, in amounts by weight equivalent to those used in vaccines, sacrificed them as young adults at eight weeks of age, and found major brain damage in all of them, including

1. ischemic degeneration of neurons in the hippocampus, cerebellum, and prefrontal and temporal cortices;

2. atrophy of glial cells in the hippocampus and cerebellum; and
3. degenerative changes in the accompanying blood vessels.[5]

A group of biochemists from the same university discovered that the brains of infant rats injected with thimerosal showed microscopic damage resembling that seen in autism, and dangerous excesses of glutamate and aspartate,[6] key amino acid derivatives that in physiologic doses function as excitatory neurotransmitters in brain tissue.[7]

Notwithstanding a prolonged campaign by the CDC to convince the public that thimerosal is harmless, the evidence against it was sufficiently compelling to persuade the European Union to remove it from all vaccines; and in 1999, the United States reluctantly followed suit. In the industrialized world, it survives only in multi-dose vials of the inactivated flu vaccine, and in trace amounts in the DTaP; but it is still widely used in Third World countries that cannot afford the latest, most expensive products and have little choice but to stop vaccinating altogether or accept whatever inferior and outdated rejects the industry dumps on them.

ALUMINUM ADJUVANTS

Aluminum is among the oldest and by far the most common adjuvant used in vaccines, occurring in 18 of the 32 now marketed for general use in the United States,[8] and it appears to be essential for them to mount an adequate immune response. The neurotoxicity of the aluminum salts found in adjuvants is also well-known and has been described for many decades. In 1965, for example, aluminum phosphate injected into the brains of rabbits was shown to produce neurofibrillary tangles and other histological changes in nerve cells that closely resemble the characteristic lesions of Alzheimer's disease.[9]

Similarly, even animals fed aluminum salts in amounts comparable to those in baking powder, antacids, and the aluminum cookware residues commonly ingested by humans were prone to developing impairments in learning, memory, and concentration, as well as confusion and repetitive behaviors.[10] But only a tiny fraction of ingested aluminum is absorbed into the blood, and even that is readily excreted in the urine,[11] whereas nearly all of the aluminum administered by injection appears in the circulation without delay[12] and is designed to remain in the body for as long as possible. For that reason, the vaccine-adjuvant complexes are molecules of high molecular weight, far larger than the kidneys are able to filter from the blood and reliably excrete.[13]

Most important of all, both aluminum salts and the vaccine-adjuvant complexes formed from them readily cross the blood-brain barrier. When labeled with the radioactive isotope aluminum-26, for example, and injected into adult female rabbits, the vaccine adjuvants aluminum hydroxide and aluminum phosphate appeared in the blood almost immediately, remained at high levels throughout the 28 days of the experiment, and were found in excessive amounts thereafter in the brain, liver, spleen, lymph nodes, and elsewhere.[14]

The aluminum-adjuvanted vaccines hepatitis A, B, and tetanus toxoid have also been implicated in the syndrome known as macrophagic myofasciitis, or MMF, consisting of muscle and joint pains and intense chronic fatigue simulating chronic fatigue syndrome (CFS), with muscle weakness and neurologic impairment, including multiple sclerosis.[15] In these patients, muscle biopsies showed extensive infiltration by macrophages and lymphocytes and damage to muscle fibers,[16] while blood tests revealed autoantibodies and high levels of the inflammatory cytokines interleukin (IL)-1 and interleukin (IL)-6.[17]

Its symptoms are remarkably similar to those of Gulf War syndrome, which has been linked to the aluminum-adjuvanted anthrax vaccine, and likewise includes degeneration of motor neurons.[18]

Moreover, the hexavalent aluminum-adjuvanted vaccines Hexavac and Infanrix Hexa have both been associated with infant death within 48 hours of injection;[19] and postmortem examination of six such cases revealed major neurodegenerative changes, including breakdown of the blood-brain barrier, diffuse congestion and infiltration of the pons, midbrain, cerebral cortex, and meninges by macrophages and T-lymphocytes, microglial proliferation in the pons and hippocampus, and necrosis of the cerebellum,[20] as well as high levels of eosinophils and mast-cell tryptase in the serum, indicating acute anaphylaxis.[21] Spurred on by these findings, the same authors discovered a 13-fold increase in infant deaths following the introduction of these hexavalent vaccines.[22]

Activation of inflammatory cytokines and other chronic inflammatory responses have long been described and identified as causal factors in Alzheimer's disease,[23] autism,[24] multiple sclerosis,[25] and the dementia seen in patients on kidney dialysis,[26] neurodegenerative diseases that have all been linked to aluminum exposure.[27,28,29,30]

Finally, the inflammatory and excitatory mechanisms elucidated for aluminum-adjuvanted vaccines are remarkably similar to those described for thimerosal, including interference with oxidative phosphorylation in the mitochondria of affected cells.[31] The overriding sense from all this research that autism represents essentially a poisoning by foreign chemicals was further confirmed by a French team, which found markedly elevated concentrations of various porphyrins, well-known biomarkers of environmental toxicity, in the urine of autistic children.[32]

As if even all that were insufficient, several years are required for young children to develop an efficient blood-brain barrier, such that the immature brains of newborns and infants are especially permeable to neurotoxins such as thimerosal and aluminum and thus at maximum risk for brain damage from vaccines. In the United States and other developed countries, infants up to six months of age receive anywhere from 14.7 to 49 times more aluminum from vaccines than the FDA's own safety limits allow,[33] while newborns in the United States, the United Kingdom, Canada, and Australia receive an amount equivalent to 10 adult hepatitis B vaccinations in a single day.[34] By two months of age they receive the equivalent of 34 adult hepatitis B vaccinations each time they go in for their shots.[35]

In an exhaustive review of the literature on aluminum toxicity,[36] Lucija Tomljenovic and Christopher Shaw, two neuroscientists at the University of British Columbia, have compiled and reviewed not only the studies I have just cited, for which I am greatly in their debt, but many more besides. Here is their summary of this hot topic in contemporary neuroscience, in words that recall the prophetic warnings of Dr. Buttram from decades ago:

> Persistent stimulation of Th2 [helper T-cells that stimulate antibody production], due to repeated administration of aluminum-adjuvanted vaccines, may have profound, long-term, adverse effects on the developing immune system in children.
>
> A newborn infant has an undeveloped immune system which is limited in function and requires a series of challenges to bring it to full capacity. Prior to the introduction of vaccines, these were largely in the form of relatively minor childhood diseases, such as mumps and measles.
>
> Vaccines stimulating antibody production by the humoral immune system (Th2), located in the bone marrow, bypass the cellular immune system (Th1) on mucosal surfaces of the respiratory and GI tracts, leaving the latter unchallenged during their critical period of development. The end result of a prolonged Th2 shift may be permanently stunted Th1 [or cellular] immunity, which is far more efficient than Th2 [the humoral system] in clearing viral pathogens.[37]

AUTOIMMUNE MECHANISMS AS THE BASIS OF VACCINE ACTION

We have seen that autoimmune phenomena, including proliferation of inflammatory cytokines and excitatory neurotransmitters, blocking oxidative phosphorylation in mitochondria, and circulating autoantibodies in blood and brain tissue, keep popping up in every kind of adverse reaction to vaccines, and to thimerosal and aluminum adjuvants all by themselves, seemingly wherever we take the trouble to look for them.

In their collection, *Vaccines & Autoimmunity,* Shoenfeld, Agmon-Levin, and Tomljenovic summarize the evidence that autoimmune phenomena can progress silently for many months or years before manifesting clinically as a disease, often in response to further environmental challenges, such as a subsequent vaccination or chemical exposure:

> We have recently reported a new syndrome, ASIA, the Autoimmune/Autoinflammatory Syndrome Induced by Adjuvants, which encompasses a spectrum of immune-mediated diseases triggered by a stimulus such as aluminum and other adjuvants, and which has also been found to induce autoimmune and inflammatory manifestations by themselves, both in animal models and in humans.
>
> In 1982, epidemiological, clinical, and animal research showed that Guillain-Barré syndrome and other demyelinating, autoimmune neuropathies, such as acute disseminated encephalomyelitis and multiple sclerosis, could occur up to ten months following vaccination.
>
> In such cases, the disease would first manifest with vague symptoms, like arthralgias, myalgias, paresthesias, and weakness, which were frequently deemed insignificant and ignored by the treating physicians. These would progress slowly and insidiously until the patient was exposed to a secondary immune stimulus, an infection or vaccination, which would then trigger the acute disease. It was the secondary response that would bring about the overt manifestation of an already present but subclinical, long-term, persistent disease.
>
> A typical vaccine formulation contains all the necessary biochemical components to induce autoimmune manifestations.[38]

The ubiquity of these subclinical phenomena, and the prolonged time lag often required for them to develop into overt disease, provide conclusive evidence for the inadequacy of the ACIP guidelines, whose stringent time limits have arbitrarily excluded almost all chronic autoimmune diseases from the list of vaccine-related complications, as we saw:

> Postmarketing surveillance is self-reported, and the reports are often incomplete, since the subject may not recognize an adverse event that is not included in the data sheet and may be distant from the time of vaccination. There are concerns that such vaccinations may be a trigger for adverse events of an autoimmune nature that manifest as a clinically recognizable disease only many months or years after administration.[39]

In a similar vein, the bulk of *Vaccines & Autoimmunity* provides evidence linking both individual vaccines to a variety of autoimmune diseases, and familiar autoimmune diseases to the vaccines that are so far known to have caused them. Regarding the MMR, for example, the autoimmune diseases so far linked to it include the following:[40]

Aseptic meningitis
Guillain-Barré syndrome
Thrombocytopenic purpura
Hemolytic anemia
Sensorineural hearing loss
Acute disseminated encephalomyelitis
Optic neuritis
Hemolytic-uremic syndrome
Acute and chronic arthritis

With the hepatitis B vaccine, the documented autoimmune diseases are exceptionally numerous and diverse:[41]

Multiple sclerosis
Myelitis
Optic neuritis
Guillain-Barré syndrome
Neuropathy
Myopathy
Myasthenia gravis
Chronic fatigue syndrome
Systemic lupus (SLE)
Antiphospholipid syndrome
Thrombocytopenia
Pancytopenia
Juvenile dermatomyositis
Still's disease
Arthritis
Vasculitis
Pulmonary vasculitis
Polyarteritis nodosa
Henoch-Schönlein purpura
Kawasaki disease
Bullous pemphigoid
Gulf War syndrome
Lichen planus
Erythema multiforme
Alopecia
Graves' disease
Glomerulonephritis

Taken together, the two HPV vaccines—Merck's Gardasil and GSK's Cervarix—account for a shocking 42% of all adverse vaccine reactions reported to the VAERS system, as well as 66% of all serious reactions, 66% of all that were life-threatening, 62% of all deaths, 80% of those resulting in permanent disability, and 72.5% of those requiring prolonged hospitalization,[42] a truly astonishing track record. These totals encompassed the following inflammatory, autoimmune diseases:[43]

Hemiparesis	Acute disseminated encephalomyelitis
Multiple sclerosis	Choreoathetosis
Unspecified demyelinating disease	Optic neuritis
Opsoclonus-myoclonus syndrome	Vascultis
Primary ovarian failure	Autoimmune pancreatitis
Thrombocytopenic purpura	Autoimmune hepatitis
Antiphospholipid syndrome	Systemic lupus (SLE)
Orthostatic tachycardia syndrome	

For the influenza vaccine, the list is as follows:[44]

Microscopic polyangiitis	Guillain-Barré syndrome
Leucocytoclastic vasculitis	Lambert-Eaton myasthenic syndrome
Henoch-Schönlein purpura	Multiple sclerosis
Temporal arteritis	Acute disseminated encephalomyelitis
Systemic lupus (SLE)	Narcolepsy
Thrombocytopenic purpura	Juvenile arthritis
Inflammatory myopathy	Still's disease

In the case of the pneumococcal vaccine, the types of autoimmune diseases linked to vaccines are rather different, albeit with some overlap:

Thrombocytopenic purpura	Hairy-cell leukemia
Bronchiectasis and COPD	Rheumatoid arthritis
Prostate adenocarcinoma	Autoimmune hemolytic anemia
Immunoblastic lymphadenopathy[45]	

In the next section, important and well-known autoimmune diseases are linked back to the several vaccines that are so far known to have caused them. The antiphospholipid syndrome is particularly relevant in this respect, since myelin, the substance lining and insulating many nerve fibers in the brain and peripheral nervous system, is a major phospholipid-protein complex, and autoantibodies directed against it are important factors in demyelinating diseases like multiple sclerosis and Guillain-Barré syndrome, and thus help explain the striking preponderance of brain and nervous-system pathology in adverse reactions caused by vaccines.[46]

All of these discoveries provide further confirmation of my own clinical experience of caring for vaccinated children and adults of all ages, that the extensive array of autoimmune phenomena caused by vaccines are not rare aberrations, but indeed are built into their design and present often enough to be the rule rather than the exception, even when the patient feels well and has no symptoms for weeks and months afterwards.

Some scientists have argued that autoimmune phenomena are ubiquitous but harmless unless the patient is pathologically hypersensitive to them, a view naturally favored by the vaccine industry and its adherents who routinely insist, as we have seen, that what appear to be adverse events are solely attributable to the genetic predispositions of the victim, such that the contribution of vaccines, herbicides, and other toxins is purely "coincidental."

As put forth by the Autoimmune Research Center at Johns Hopkins, the more balanced, more plausible, and indeed more typical explanation is that autoimmune responses involve *both* preexisting susceptibility *and* exposure to environmental agents, just as Shoenfeld and his colleagues have been documenting and insisting upon:

> The healthy body is equipped with powerful tools for resisting invading microorganisms, known as the immune system, which sometimes goes awry and attacks the body itself. These misdirected responses, known as autoimmunity, can be demonstrated by the presence of autoantibodies or T-lymphocytes reactive with host antigens.
>
> Autoimmunity is present in everyone to some extent. It is usually harmless and probably a universal phenomenon of vertebrate life. However, it can also cause a broad spectrum of human illnesses, known as autoimmune diseases. These are defined as diseases in which benign autoimmunity progresses to a pathogenic type, which is determined by genetic influences and environmental triggers.[47]

Both to tease out how autoimmune diseases might develop from at first or seemingly harmless responses, and to investigate the possibility that autoimmune processes are the basis for how vaccines work, a simple first step might be to track serum titers of C-reactive protein, erythrocyte sedimentation rate, and other well-known markers in both vaccinated and unvaccinated patients, and to be more attentive to vague, nondescript symptoms as possible early warning signs of autoimmunity, rather than waiting until they blossom into overt, full-blown disease.

In another example of promising scientific work that has been largely ignored, it turns out that a group of veterinarians at Purdue University carried out just such an experiment in the late 1990s, with remarkable results. Two groups of five purebred beagle puppies, one vaccinated on the schedule typical for pet dogs and the other unvaccinated, were followed closely for three years, with a series of blood tests and immunoassays. Although none of the dogs in their small sample developed overt clinical disease during that time, every one of the vaccinated group demonstrated significant titers of autoantibodies directed against important tissue proteins, chiefly

1. fibronectin, antibodies against which are significantly implicated in the pathogenesis of scleroderma, rheumatoid arthritis, and systemic lupus in dogs, humans, and other species;
2. laminin, antibodies against which are found in rheumatoid arthritis, lupus, glomerulonephritis, and vasculitis;
3. cardiolipin, implicated in cardiomyopathy, and
4. cytochrome C, collagen, transferrin, serum albumin and DNA,

while none of the unvaccinated dogs did so.[48] Furthermore, the same authors were able to show that

> These proteins are typically of bovine origin, since fetal calf serum is used to grow the viruses for vaccine production. Their close similarity to dog proteins results in a situation where antibodies produced by vaccinated dogs may cross-react with dog tissue proteins in a process similar to autoimmunity.
>
> Experiments in other species suggest that these autoantibodies might eventually cause diseases in the vaccinated animals. These beagles will have to be followed longer to determine if this is the case. In addition, the pattern of individual responses suggests a possible genetic predisposition to auto-immunity.
>
> The above study is unique in its attempt to determine if routine vaccinations received throughout life have a cumulative adverse effect. The only way this is possible is if one group of dogs remains unvaccinated.[49]

Sadly, the authors' clear recommendation that the study period be extended was never heeded by the university or given sufficient funding to be carried out, as far as I'm aware.

OTHER VACCINE INGREDIENTS

So far, as we have seen, most experimental work has been devoted to the adverse effects of aluminum adjuvants and thimerosal, both of which have been known for generations to be highly toxic to many different tissues and organ systems, and to the brain and nervous system predominantly, a specificity that closely parallels the anatomical distribution of adverse reactions to vaccines generally.

But such studies are not directly applicable to live-virus vaccines, such as MMR, varicella, and rotavirus, which exhibit similar patterns of toxicity without any need for aluminum or mercury. Nor have they investigated the large number and extensive array of other foreign substances in vaccines, some of which are known to be toxic, while others, seemingly innocuous by themselves, in their diverse combinations might not be. The CDC's repeated assurances that all of these ingredients are safe are hardly persuasive or even credible, since they fail to provide any evidence of the slightest attempt to investigate them.

Here follows a very partial listing of some other ingredients that happened to catch my eye:

Formaldehyde

Used to inactivate and kill the parent microorganisms of the DTaP, Hep B, Hib, influenza, meningococcus, and polio vaccines, formaldehyde is a potent carcinogen, while in the amounts used it has also been shown to generate reactive carbonyl groups that further boost the intended Th2 responses to these vaccines, and to promote other viral infections upon subsequent exposure.[50] By any estimate, it is clearly a dangerous chemical; and as a component of vaccines it deserves far more careful scrutiny than it has so far received.

Glutaraldehyde

Another transient aldehyde formed in the physiological degradation of the normal amino acid lysine, glutaraldehyde is used as a disinfectant to clean medical and lab equipment, and has been linked to a variety of allergic and hypersensitivity responses, including asthma,[51] and clearly warrants further investigation of its precise role and mechanism of action in vaccines, chiefly the DTaP.

2-Phenoxyethanol

A phenylether derivative of ethylene glycol, or antifreeze, 2-phenoxyethanol is a preservative and disinfectant used in the DTaP and polio vaccines as an alternative to thimerosal. It has been shown to inhibit the glutamate and aspartate receptors in the brain tissue of experimental animals, leading to impaired memory and learning capacity, altered sensory processing, ataxia, and various other neurological disturbances, as well as vacuolation and other neuropathological changes.[52]

Other phenolated hydrocarbons, such as nonyl- and octylphenol ethoxylate and phenol itself, antiseptics and germicides with serious toxic potential, are also used in some influenza vaccines, and certainly warrant further scrutiny.

Polysorbate 80 and Other Emulsifiers

Included as an emulsifier in the DTaP, HPV, influenza, pneumococcus, and rotavirus vaccines, the detergent polysorbate 80 is a polymer of ethylene oxide and oleic acid that acts as a surfactant in foods, cosmetics, and household cleaners. Since it is known and indeed widely used to facilitate the transport of various drugs and chemotherapeutic agents across the blood-brain barrier,[53] the obvious question that nobody seems to be asking is whether it might be acting synergistically with aluminum, mercury, and the other known neurotoxins to provide even easier access to the brain of infants and children especially, and thus add to their already high risk of autism and other forms of brain damage.

Like polysorbate 80, the bile salts sodium deoxycholate and taurodeoxycholate are used as detergents and emulsifying agents in influenza vaccines, similarly render the blood-brain barrier more permeable to various drugs,[54] and thus pose comparable risks of added neurotoxicity.

Antibiotics

The antibiotics neomycin, polymyxin B, gentamicin, and kanamycin are added to influenza and polio vaccines to prevent bacterial contamination. Even in small amounts, they could promote the emergence of resistant strains, and therefore merit careful study.

Animal Cell Lines from Tissue Culture

The following cellular and protein extracts from animals and microbial sources are components of almost all vaccines:

Cell Lines[55]	**Vaccines**
Fetal lung tissue	Varicella, Shingles
Fetal diploid lung fibroblasts	MMR
Monkey kidney cells	Polio (IPV)
Chick embryo cell culture	MMR
Yeast cells	Pneumococcus

Proteins and Cell Extracts[56]	**Vaccines**
Fetal bovine serum	MMR, Rotavirus, Varicella
Bovine calf serum	Polio, Shingles
Bovine extract	DTaP
Insect cell and viral protein	HPV
Yeast protein	Hep B, HPV
Egg protein	Influenza
Gelatin	DTaP, Influenza, Varicella

Although the safety of injecting these cells and extracts has not yet been investigated carefully, as far as I know, and I'm unaware of any definite evidence linking them to serious disease, nobody has ever plausibly explained how mainlining foreign cells, DNA, and protein antigens directly into the bloodstream could *fail* to elicit a significant harvest of immune and autoimmune responses all by themselves; and the CDC's deafening silence on the matter is hardly reassuring. If they can prove them to be innocuous, wholesome, and health-giving, no one will be happier than I; but the public surely deserves an honest accounting of the evidence. Here are the doubts, fears, and ruminations of Dr. Palevsky, the pediatrician we've met before, on the unexamined menace of these foreign antigenic ingredients:

> A virus is not "alive" *per se*; it's simply a strand of RNA or DNA, and by itself can't "do" anything. In addition, it's so tiny that it's much smaller than bacteria, and can only be seen under an electron microscope. So they can't be isolated

> when you make a vaccine of them; all that can be isolated is the tissue, whether human or animal, believed to have been infected by it.
>
> When viral cultures are made, you're going to have the DNA of people or animals who were already infected. Those cells are then taken and grown on animal cells, like monkey kidney or chicken embryo cells. When mixed together, these cells will splice and recombine, so that DNA from animal cells mixes with DNA from the cells known to have been infected with the virus. So by definition, a viral vaccine contains foreign animal and possibly human DNA.
>
> The question is, how safe is it to inject viral material that is embedded into the DNA of foreign cells? What studies have been done to test if foreign DNA is actually getting into your body, if it stays in your DNA, if it gets into your brain, and if there are foreign animal viruses that are already present in animal DNA to begin with?[57]

It is profoundly shocking that no independent scientific investigation of these materials has ever been undertaken; but it seems highly probable, if not virtually certain, that large numbers of people have already been harmed by them, and will continue to be in the future, just as they would be from blood transfusions and organ transplants from different species, as in effect they are.

Contaminants

In addition to the various inbred cell lines, natural and artificial culture media, and the complex techniques employed for propagating them, the preparation of vaccines poses still other health risks, both known and unknown, by no means the least of which is contamination with other viruses.

To date, by far the most important and scandalous example was SV40, a cancer-causing virus native to monkeys that found its way into the original injectable polio vaccine (IPV), and was inadvertently injected into about 10 million to 30 million American infants and children, by the CDC's own estimate, between 1955 and 1963, when it was identified and removed.[58] Nor can anyone guarantee that it won't reappear in the future, or that it hasn't already done so, in either or both versions of the vaccine.

Since then, SV40 has been reliably linked to mesothelioma, a type of lung cancer also caused by asbestos; to medulloblastoma, an especially deadly form of brain cancer; to several types of bone cancer; and to thousands of deaths from various other types of cancer in the United States and elsewhere.[59]

Another such contaminant is porcine circovirus, two subtypes of which have been identified in the rotavirus vaccines,[60] but not as yet linked to any specific disease. While a number of scientists have gone so far as to claim that *all* vaccines are contaminated, I will simply repeat the words of Dr. Philip Krause, a senior scientist at the FDA, who is certainly in a position to know:

> In the past, biologic products have served as vectors for viral diseases. Examples include the contamination of Yellow Fever vaccine with the Hepatitis B virus in the 1940s, from a human-derived excipient; contamination of early polio and adenovirus vaccines with SV40 in the late 1950s and early 1960s, contamination of donated blood with Hepatitis and AIDS viruses, and contamination of dura mater grafts with the Creitzfeldt-Jakob or Mad Cow Disease agent.
>
> Production of viral vaccines involves inoculation of a cell substrate with a vaccine seed and purification of bulk product from these cells after sufficient time for replication of the virus or production of vaccine proteins. Other raw materials (e.g., tissue culture reagents, stabilizers) may be added at various stages. Adventitious agents could enter a vaccine through any of these ingredients.[61]

Culture Media

Finally, the parent microorganisms of many vaccines must first be grown and propagated on various culture media, which may contain not only the cell lines already described, but also a bewildering array of nutrients and buffers, many of which appear innocuous enough in themselves, but might not be in proximity to or chemical combination with the rest. Without attempting to provide a complete list, I will mention a few, to give some idea of the number and complexity of the substances involved:

- **Stainer-Scholte Medium** (in DTaP): monosodium glutamate (MSG), potassium chloride, potassium phosphate, sodium chloride, magnesium chloride, calcium chloride, ferrous sulfate, vitamins, and glutathione;
- **Muller-Miller Medium** (in Hib, meningococcus): glucose, sodium and potassium phosphates, magnesium sulfate, ferrous sulfate, amino acids, uracil, sodium hydroxide, beef heart, and casein;
- **Soy Peptone Broth** (in Hep B, influenza, pneumococcus): amino acids from soy protein, digested with papain, a proteolytic enzyme;
- **Monosodium Glutamate,** or MSG (in DTaP, influenza, varicella, shingles);

- **Urea** (in varicella);
- **Ammonium Sulfate** (in Hib, pneumococcus);
- **Beta-Propiolactone,** a known carcinogen[62] (in influenza, rotavirus); and
- **Hydrocortisone** (in influenza).[63]

Once again, these various substances and combinations are generally thought to be required for culturing, preparing, and stabilizing the vaccines, as no doubt they are; but the rules for using chemical substances in artificial media have very little to do with the rules that need to be followed before injecting them into the blood and brains of millions of little children, let alone mandating them into law. It beggars the imagination that we still allow matters of such importance to remain lucrative trade secrets of an industry that has enjoyed a virtual *carte blanche* over our public health for these many decades.

SUMMARY

In our review of basic science research on vaccines, we have focused on three main topics:

1. the autoimmune mechanisms for the toxicity of vaccines containing the preservative thimerosal and various soluble aluminum salts as adjuvants, and for their neurotoxicity in particular;
2. autoimmunity as the basic pathway of virtually all adverse reactions to vaccines that have so far been identified; and
3. the still largely unknown and seldom investigated health risks of the myriad of other vaccine ingredients.

In amounts found in vaccines, the preservative thimerosal and various aluminum adjuvants have both been shown to damage brain tissue especially, as well as organs and tissues in every other part of the body, by essentially the same mechanism, namely, hypersecretion of interleukins (inflammatory cytokines) and the excitatory neurotransmitters glutamate and aspartate, which promote autoimmune inflammation and infiltration by lymphocytes and macrophages, interrupt aerobic energy production in the mitochondria, and ultimately can result in brain damage, whether in the form of autism, encephalopathy, or demyelinating and degenerative diseases.

The brain is especially vulnerable to this kind of damage, because both thimerosal and aluminum salts readily cross the blood-brain barrier, especially in infants, and because the brain is entirely dependent on aerobic mechanisms for its energy, accounting for only 2% of the body by weight, but consuming fully 20% of its oxygen.

The work of Shoenfeld, Tomljenovic, and their colleagues have highlighted autoimmune mechanisms in a wide variety of adverse vaccine reactions and the extensive array of autoimmune diseases that can ultimately ensue. Their recognition of the so-called ASIA syndrome, the autoimmune syndrome induced by adjuvants, provided clear proof that adverse reactions to vaccines may begin subclinically, and often require months or years, and possibly additional vaccine challenges, before they become diagnosable or even develop symptoms, in any case well beyond the CDC's strict time limit for any ongoing chronic disease to be accepted as vaccine-related.

These findings cry out for revision of these unrealistic guidelines, for developing methods of identifying susceptible individuals in advance, and for safer vaccines that are sensitive to these differences, rather than persisting in the reckless strategy of "one size fits all."

The final section includes a survey of the vast and truly bewildering array of other vaccine ingredients, almost all of which have remained "trade secrets" of the industry, carefully protected from public scrutiny, yet still rubber-stamped by the CDC and virtually the whole of the medical profession, in spite of legitimate concerns and doubts about their safety.

Even a quick look at the list is like opening a veritable Pandora's box of health hazards, some already known, others quite probable, and all deserving further study, including

1. *known carcinogens* such as formaldehyde and beta-propiolactone;
2. *allergens* such as glutaraldehyde;
3. *aromatic hydrocarbons,* including phenol and 2-phenoxyethanol;
4. *detergents* such as polysorbate 80 and bile salts, which are used to emulsify drugs and vaccines and may deliberately or inadvertently help them cross the blood-brain barrier;
5. *antibiotics;*
6. *foreign animal cell lines used in tissue culture* (e.g., from monkey kidneys, insects, aborted human fetuses, bovine cell extracts, fertilized chicken embryos, *and various serums and protein antigens derived from them*);

7. *contaminants* such as the simian virus SV40, already a major cause of cancer (albeit recognized and supposedly eliminated long ago), porcine circoviruses, and doubtless others as yet unidentified; and
8. *culture media,* containing chemicals such as MSG, ammonium sulfate, and hydrocortisone, as well as phosphate, sulfate, and chloride salts and buffers, largely innocuous in themselves, but maybe not in the combination.

My hope and fervent prayer is that the medical profession and the scientific community will recognize the hazard of these chemicals, and that the general public will persuade them to carry out detailed investigations and make the data readily accessible to everyone.

PART IV

THE INDIVIDUAL VACCINES

Chapter 11

THE BIG THREE

In the next three chapters, I will consider the vaccines individually, together with the natural diseases that they correspond to and are directed against.

THE DPT, DTP, AND DTAP

Diphtheria and tetanus toxoids have been in use since the 1920s; the pertussis vaccine, containing an emulsion of the heat-killed bacterium *Bordetella pertussis*, was added in the late 1940s, by which time all three diseases were already declining rapidly in both prevalence and morbidity. Originally known as the DPT, the new triple vaccine became the DTP in the 1990s, and finally the DTaP in the early 2000s, with the development of the acellular pertussis component.

With vaccines mandated for school attendance on a state-by-state basis, the triple combination did not become a nationwide requirement until the late 1970s, the point at which the courts began to be inundated with lawsuits for brain damage, as we saw, with momentous consequences that are still very much with us today, including

1. the 1986 Act of Congress that created the Vaccine Adverse Event Reporting System and the Vaccine Injury Compensation Program, and
2. the nationwide movement of parents advocating for safer vaccines, more regulation of the industry, and more transparency on the part of the CDC.

Although never fully acknowledged by the CDC's Advisory Committee on Immunization Practices, the history of "DPT encephalopathy"—a form of brain damage—and of SIDS and other varieties of infant death occurring after vaccination, have already been described in detail, and need no further elaboration here.

As to its effectiveness or lack thereof, I will say more presently; but the outcry occasioned by these lawsuits and the quasi-legal mechanism designed to supersede them unquestionably prompted development of the somewhat safer acellular pertussis vaccine as well. One memorable tidbit of this history was the report of an official task force commissioned by the American Academy of Pediatrics, and headed by Dr. James Cherry, a leading vaccine advocate, which admitted that Japan's policy of postponing both whole-cell and acellular DPT vaccinations until 24 months of age caused the disappearance of SIDS as a public health issue in that country;[1] yet such is the reverence accorded to the vaccination concept in the United States that neither Dr. Cherry nor any of his colleagues ever saw fit to recommend or even contemplate such a plan here.

From the beginning, all versions of the DPT vaccine have used aluminum adjuvants; in addition to aluminum hydroxide, the DTaP also contains the detergent polysorbate 80, the germicides formaldehyde and glutaraldehyde, and foreign proteins, namely, bovine extract and bovine casein.[2] The neurotoxicity of vaccines adjuvanted with aluminum salts has already been detailed, with the added risk of polysorbate 80 helping them cross the blood-brain barrier even more readily, yet another small, technical detail that hasn't been talked about, but certainly should be.

Pertussis

In 1942, when the whole-cell vaccine was first introduced, both the incidence and severity of pertussis had already declined dramatically, thanks largely to improvements in sanitation and general health, to an extent that epidemiologists were highly skeptical that future decreases could reasonably be credited to the vaccine,[3] as we saw. In 1977, Professor Gordon Stewart of Glasgow University in Scotland went even further, citing its known risks as reason enough to invalidate the rationale for using it, and providing a simple, rough-and-ready criterion for evaluating any vaccine that remains highly pertinent even today: "This risk [of DPT encephalopathy] far exceeds the present risk of death or permanent damage from whooping-cough, or even, in some parts of the country, from the chance of contracting it."[4]

In short, the substantial risk of brain damage, which later research into the aluminum-containing vaccines has shown to be far more prevalent than in his early estimate, already demonstrated that the vaccine lacked any practical usefulness when compared to simply letting the disease continue to fade away at its own rapid and steady pace. A subsequent article by Professor Stewart made the same point even more forcefully, by pointing out that whooping cough had already become a relatively mild disease in most cases, and that recovery from it also provided lifelong immunity, which vaccination clearly did not:

> In the UK and many other countries, whooping cough and measles are no longer important causes of death or severe illness, except in a small minority of infants who are otherwise disadvantaged. I cannot see how it is justifiable to promote mass vaccination of children everywhere against diseases which are generally mild, confer lasting immunity, and which are easily overcome by most children without being vaccinated.[5]

In any case, the strategy of vaccinating everyone has predictably backfired in a major way, by ending and indeed reversing this wholly favorable trend.

Pertussis Cases in the United States[6]	
1930	166,914
1940	183,866
1950	120,718
1960	14,809
1970	4,249
1980	1,730
1985	3,589
1990	4,570
1995	7,796
2000	7,867
2005	25,616
2010	27,550
2012	48,277

With the specter of brain damage from the DPT and DTP looming greater and greater, the development of the acellular vaccine, directed against specific proteins of the bacterium, has also hastened the emergence of resistant strains lacking these antigens,[7] as well as an entirely different species, *Bordetella parapertussis*,[8] both of which have contributed to a dramatic resurgence of a generally more virulent form of the disease in recent years, with extensive outbreaks occurring in highly vaccinated populations, and even public health officials admitting for the first time that asymptomatic, vaccinated carriers are mainly responsible for the transmission,[9] rather than the unvaccinated kids who have always taken the blame for it in the past.

Diphtheria and Tetanus

Developed in the 1920s, the diphtheria and tetanus toxoids were not meant to prevent infections by these bacteria, but simply to antidote the deadly poisons elaborated by them, both of which are proteins of high molecular weight, microgram-for-microgram among the most lethal substances known to man, and are responsible for the high mortality rate of these diseases, which even today, with the best treatment available, still approaches 10%. It is thus wholly understandable that most of the parents whose children I care for in my practice have welcomed whatever protection these toxoids can provide, many of whom opt for the DT, polio, and nothing else.

In spite of broad consensus among the scientific community that, as with pertussis, these diseases were already very much on the wane in the United States before their toxoids were mandated for everyone in the 1980s, it is highly probable that the latter have played at least a substantial part in that decline. If so, that is an achievement that the industry and the medical community can rightfully be proud of.

In the case of diphtheria, for example, the CDC records 206,000 cases in 1922 and an average of only 1.67 cases per year in the period from 1980 through 2014, although scattered, small-scale outbreaks still occur from time to time.[10] Now that the toxin has been shown to be elaborated mainly by strains of the organism harboring a certain bacteriophage, or parasitic virus,[11] it is very likely that mild, non-toxicogenic cases of the disease are also continuing to occur, and that most of them go unrecognized and unreported, as they always have.

Tetanus, on the other hand, has never been common. A CDC graph shows an incidence of a little over 3 per 100,000 in 1900,[12] when the total US population was about 76 million,[13] which would add up to approximately 2,400 cases per year. Like diphtheria and pertussis, it too had been declining precipitously well before the toxoid came into wide use in the late 1940s, perhaps, in part, as a result of its notable success in preventing the disease among the US Armed

Forces in World War II. In the period from 1980 through 2014, it continued to decline as follows:

Years	Average Cases/Year
1980–89	72
1990–99	41
2000–09	29
2010–14	30[14]

From its excellent record on battlefields all over the world, where the organism would have been especially prevalent and those exposed to it highly vulnerable on account of their wounds, it is reasonable to conclude that tetanus toxoid has been effective in the general population as well.

On the other hand, both toxoids are denatured with formaldehyde; and it is well documented that death, brain damage, and serious autoimmune reactions can and do occur in highly sensitive individuals after receiving them. Although it is reasonable to suppose that these tragedies are somewhat less frequent than for the other vaccines to be considered, it is difficult to be precise about it, because in small children at least the toxoids are typically given with pertussis in the triple DTaP vaccine, of which the pertussis component is by far the main culprit; and the adult dose of the toxoid, even for an actual wound, is usually given as the DT, in combination with diphtheria, despite being available separately.

Tetanus is also in a special category because the disease cannot be transmitted from person to person and was never common to begin with; the conditions required for it to develop are so exacting and so well-known that proper wound hygiene will prevent it, and indeed has prevented it in all but a few dozen cases each year, vaccine or no vaccine. It is an extremely fastidious bacterium that can thrive only under strictly anaerobic conditions (i.e., in the total absence of oxygen).

Clostridium tetani lives mainly in the intestinal tract of horses, where it propagates itself by forming spores; these are excreted in the manure. When thus deposited in the soil and exposed to the air, tetanus spores are remarkably resistant to extremes of heat and cold, and can survive intact for decades, germinating only in oxygen-free environments—i.e., either a deep and jagged puncture wound that produces sufficient tissue damage for the organism to feed on and then closes over, sealing it off from the air; or an open wound that becomes infected, like the umbilical-cord stump of a newborn baby, where the local bacteria utilize all the available oxygen, leaving the spores free to germinate underneath them.

In short, even when the spores are present, careful wound hygiene—and above all not allowing the wound to close until it is thoroughly cleaned out—will ordinarily prevent them from germinating. Although it makes perfect sense to use the toxoid in battlefield conditions involving close combat and the inevitable likelihood of getting infected wounds, for conscientious, well-informed parents under normal conditions of civilized life, it is almost always unnecessary.

Since most parents still want it anyway, just to be on the safe side, my advice to them is simply to wait as long as possible, at least until the children are three years old, say, by which time their immune systems will have been developing normally—that is, coming down with and recovering from fevers and acute illnesses on their own, before vaccines begin reprogramming them to respond more chronically to microbes, allergens, and everything else.

In any case, the increasing urbanization of modern life, and the progressive elimination of pasturage for horses that inevitably accompanies it, seem destined to continue and further accelerate the disappearance of the disease that is already well under way.

POLIO

For reference, I'll begin with a brief excerpt from the CDC's own Polio Information Statement:

> **History**
> In 1916, a US polio epidemic killed 6,000 and paralyzed 27,000.
> In the early 1950s, over 25,000 cases were reported annually.
> In 1955, the injectable polio vaccine (IPV) was introduced.
> In 1960, only about 3,000 cases were reported.
> In 1979, only about 10 cases were reported.[15]

Although the IPV or injectable polio vaccine in current use contains no adjuvants, it does make use of several ingredients that are either known to be toxic or at least seem suspicious or questionable and deserve further investigation, namely the disinfectants and preservatives formaldehyde and 2-phenoxyethanol; the dye phenol red, and several antibiotics (streptomycin, neomycin, and polymyxin B); the complex hydrocarbon hydroxyethylpiperazine ethanesulfonic acid; Vero cells from African green monkey kidneys; and serum from newborn calves and others 3 weeks to 12 months of age.[16]

Crippling and deadly as they undoubtedly were, the legendary epidemics of paralytic poliomyelitis in 1950s America were notable for the relatively small number of deaths and long-term paralysis, and the low attack rate of the virus itself, which was ubiquitous during these epidemics, to the extent that it was found routinely in samples of city sewage wherever it was looked for.[17] Since it was impossible at the time to predict who would or would not be susceptible to it, the great microbiologist René Dubos felt it his duty to try to calm the fears that haunted my parents and virtually everyone else throughout my childhood:

> It is barely recognized but nevertheless true that animals, plants, and men can live peacefully with their most notorious microbial enemies. The world is obsessed by the fact that poliomyelitis can kill and maim several thousand unfortunate victims every year. But more extraordinary is the fact that millions upon millions of young people become infected with polioviruses, yet suffer no harm from them. The dramatic episodes of conflict between men and microbes are what strike the mind. What is less readily apprehended is the more common fact that infection can occur without producing disease.[18]

As we saw, the dramatic elimination of paralytic poliomyelitis was achieved in no small measure by the CDC's timely redefinition of the disease, neatly coinciding with the introduction of the vaccine, to apply solely to ongoing cases of paralysis lasting 60 days or more, and excluding the far more numerous cases of temporary paralysis that corrected themselves within a few days or so, which had always been counted in the past. This strategy might have been entirely legitimate and sensible had it not been devised to mislead the public by claiming that the vaccine was responsible for the decline, rather than admitting that the threat was that much less serious than previously thought and the chances of any given individual acquiring it were almost vanishingly small.

As the Nobel Prize winner Sir Macfarlane Burnet has pointed out, well over 90% of the people exposed to the poliovirus don't manifest symptoms at all, even under epidemic conditions,[19] while of the few percent who do get sick, the vast majority develop nothing more sinister than a nondescript flu-like illness with both upper respiratory tract symptoms and a gastroenteritis that is clinically indistinguishable from a host of other typical summer diarrheas in children. Of these symptomatic cases, at most 1 or 2% will progress to the full-blown picture of paralytic disease, with its typical lesions in the motor neurons of the spinal cord and brain stem;[20] and of these, the majority will resolve spontaneously in a few days, a natural history that undoubtedly helped persuade the CDC to restrict the diagnosis of paralytic polio to the tiny fraction of cases who did not.

In short, developing paralytic poliomyelitis requires a degree of anatomical susceptibility that very few people possess, one that allows the virus to migrate from the intestinal tract to the motor neurons of the spinal cord and brain stem.

As an attenuated live virus, the OPV, or oral vaccine, is subject to shedding by asymptomatic carriers, back mutations to virulence, and widely scattered, small-scale epidemics as a result, which have occurred in places as far apart as Haiti and the Dominican Republic, Nigeria, Madagascar, and the Philippines, Indonesia, and China,[21] and that ultimately led the United States and most developed countries to abandon it in favor of the original injectable Salk vaccine, or IPV, which does not prevent infection by the virus, but only its risk of attacking the nervous system.

But even though it is likely that both the oral and injectable vaccines have contributed to the further decline of the disease over the years after it was redefined, a more sensible strategy than vaccinating everybody against a disease that only a tiny fraction will ever come down with would be to elucidate the mechanism of its migration from the intestine to the spinal cord, and develop a test for identifying susceptible individuals beforehand, since even if the vaccine were completely successful in blocking polioviruses from reaching their spinal cord and brain stem, they could still be vulnerable to other viruses with the same affinity, and perhaps to complications from the vaccines themselves.

Indeed, these developments have already begun to show themselves. In the first place, the OPV or live-virus oral vaccine remains in wide use throughout much of the developing world because it is so economical, so easy to prepare, and seemingly so effective in preventing infection by the target strains of poliovirus so far identified.

But as the incidence of these strains of paralytic polio has declined, other enteroviruses and possibly even some polioviruses not covered by the vaccine have arisen to occupy the niche thus vacated; and the resulting illness, euphemistically named non-polio acute flaccid paralysis, or NPAFP, has not only become increasingly prevalent in a number of countries, but also clinically more virulent on average than polio itself. In India, for example, Vashisht and colleagues demonstrated that the incidence of NPAFP has increased dramatically between 2000 and 2013 in direct proportion to the number of doses of OPV given:

> Although the annual incidence of paralytic polio has decreased, the rate of NPAFP has increased to 11.82 per 100,000 nationwide [approximately 118,200 cases], whereas the expected rate is only 1–2 per 100,000. Follow-up of these NPAFP cases is not done routinely. However, in 2005, in the state of Uttar Pradesh, one-fifth of the cases were followed up for 60 days; 32.5% were found to have residual paralysis, and 8.5% had died [both percentages much higher than expected]. There is thus a compelling reason to determine the underlying cause for this surge in numbers.
>
> NPAFP increased with the number of OPV doses used: the rate in 2013, for example, correlated best with the cumulative doses received in the previous seven years. This correlation was highly significant; on multiple regression analysis the number of OPV doses was the only factor that showed a positive correlation with the NPAFP rate. Similarly, in Bihar and Uttar Pradesh states, where the NPAFP rate had increased every year until 2011, it declined in 2012, coinciding with a reduction in OPV doses.[22]

Moreover, a remarkably similar illness has recently broken out in the United States and been traced to enterovirus D68, suggesting that even the killed IPV can stimulate the same kind of strain and species replacement as the live OPV. The CDC has identified 120 children in 34 states who came down with a polio-like illness from August 2014 through July 2015, consisting of limb weakness or paralysis and MRI evidence of inflammation of the spinal cord.[23] Designating it as "Acute Flaccid Myelitis," they found the following additional characteristics:

1. The median age of the children was seven years.
2. Almost all were hospitalized and put on ventilators.
3. Most had fever and respiratory symptoms before CNS involvement.
4. Seventy percent had white cells and protein in their spinal fluid.
5. By day 19, 80 had improved, 40 had not, and only two had fully recovered.
6. Still, no specific virus was identified as responsible.[24]

That disclaimer may have been intended to mislead or reassure, since previous investigators had already fingered enterovirus D68 in a high percentage of such cases.[25] In any event, many other enterovirus serotypes have been identified in outbreaks of AFM (also known as acute flaccid paralysis, or AFP) from all around the world. In Shandong Province, China, for instance, a recent survey of stool samples from over 9,200 cases of AFP and over 1,000 of their contacts from

1988–2013 found over 960 of them, or almost 10%, to be positive for non-polio enteroviruses, encompassing no less than 53 different varieties.[26]

Of course, this proliferation of related viruses doesn't exactly prove that polio vaccination was the cause; but it does lend further credence to the hypothesis that massive inhibition of the three strains of poliovirus contained in both the oral and injectable vaccines has cleared a path for related strains and species to take their places in the causation of "acute flaccid paralysis" and perhaps GBS and other neurological syndromes as well, a conjecture rendered more plausible still by the CDC's studied refusal even to consider it.

As if these developments weren't enough, the greatest scandal haunting the polio vaccines arose from the unrecognized presence of the SV40 virus in the monkey kidney cells that were used as a culture medium for them; as we saw, these cells were soon found to harbor a number of other monkey viruses, whose effect on humans was and remains as yet unknown. In 1960, Dr. Bernice Eddy of the NIH found that the monkey kidney cells were dying off prematurely, that injecting them into hamsters produced tumors, and that the oncogenic factor was a virus;[27] Dr. Maurice Hillerman at Merck called it SV40, because it was the 40th simian virus to be found in that cell line alone.[28]

Unfortunately, between 1955, when the Salk vaccine was introduced, and 1960, when the virus SV40 was discovered in it, 98 million Americans, both children and adults, had already received the vaccine, and it is now estimated that between 10% and 30% of these doses had been contaminated with SV40, as well as a similar percentage for the 10 million Americans and many millions of Russians who had already received the OPV.[29]

But while SV40 had been shown to cause cancers in hamsters and other experimental animals, its possible carcinogenicity in humans remained unproven, and indeed, as we've come to expect, was stoutly resisted by the CDC, the manufacturers, and their physician-advocates. Even though the cancer rate for American children had continued to rise fairly dramatically and consistently throughout the 1960s, 1970s, 1980s, and 1990s,[30] and SV40 DNA had been detected in a variety of cancer specimens all over the world, chiefly brain tumors,[31] bone cancers,[32] and mesotheliomas,[33] the very same tumor cell types that appeared when it was injected into experimental animals,[34] both the CDC and the National Cancer Institute have persistently disputed any such link, and commissioned a number of in-house studies to disprove it.

Although SV40 was finally and reluctantly declared a Class 2A or "probable" human carcinogen in 2002, after years of official stonewalling,[35] the CDC and the industry have continued to drag their feet in the follow-through,[36] so that we still do not know precisely how many human cancers have resulted from other contaminants that may be lurking undetected.

THE MMR

A live-virus vaccine, the MMR needs no adjuvants, disinfectants, or preservatives, but does contain the antibiotic neomycin, the excitatory neurotransmitter glutamate, and a large number of foreign animal and human cells and proteins, namely, chick embryo cell culture, fetal bovine serum, WI-38 human diploid lung fibroblasts from a female fetus that was aborted in 1964, fetal bovine serum, and recombinant human albumin.[37]

Whereas the first vaccines, smallpox, DPT, and polio, were all directed against serious and potentially fatal or crippling "foreign" diseases, the MMR broke new ground in targeting three "normal diseases of childhood" that most children eventually came down with and almost all recovered from. Partly for that reason, MMR has always been one of the most controversial vaccines, and is still hotly debated by the "vaccine establishment" who promote it aggressively, on the one side, and the uncounted tens of thousands of parents, at the very least, who are convinced that it killed or damaged their children, on the other.

That it causes autism and other forms of brain and neurological impairment in very large numbers of susceptible children has already been proven beyond a reasonable doubt, as we saw, and recently verified by a senior CDC scientist who remorsefully confessed his role in the government's cover-up of its own data to that effect for at least 15 years. Nor is autism by any means the whole story of the harm the MMR has done, which includes death, Guillain-Barré syndrome (GBS), acute disseminated encephalomyelitis (ADEM), encephalopathy, epilepsy, inflammatory bowel disease, diabetes, arthritis, ITP and bleeding disorders, and a wide variety of other autoimmune diseases, including the rare, tragic case of nephrotic syndrome and permanent kidney damage that I myself was privy to. Since these adverse effects have already been surveyed in detail, I need not elaborate on them again.

But in addition to the direct harm that they do, one of the worst and least-discussed complications of the MMR, and indeed of vaccines in general, is the major health benefit that is denied or withheld when they achieve their intended purpose, the substitution of specific antibodies as an isolated technical feat for the splendid, massive, and concerted outpouring of the immune system as a whole in response to acute infections, involving both Th1 and Th2 responses working together, and culminating in expulsion of the foreign virus or bacterium from the blood.

As we saw in chapter 1, coming down with and recovering from acute illnesses with fever are the formative experiences for the normal maturation of the child's immune mechanism, resulting in both an absolute, lifelong immunity to the specific microorganism involved, and a nonspecific priming of the system to respond acutely and vigorously to whatever else may threaten it in the future, an enormous net gain for the individual and the community.

In the case of the live-virus vaccines, notably measles, mumps, rubella, and chicken pox, we have seen that these actions confer important health benefits throughout life in the form of substantial protection against a large number of major chronic diseases that vaccinated children are increasingly prone to, namely, asthma, allergies, seizures, diabetes, autoimmune diseases, degenerative diseases of the brain and nervous system, and various forms of cancer.

In place of these huge, life-affirming benefits, the best that vaccination can offer is only a somewhat lower risk of coming down with a particular acute disease, which is more than offset by the added risk of these other chronic and potentially life-threatening diseases later in life, as well as a marked predisposition to develop autoimmune reactions to other foreign substances, such as food allergies or intolerances, chemical exposures, and the like.

In addition, as with the other live-virus vaccines—oral polio, varicella, shingles, rotavirus, and inhaled influenza—the fundamental mystery remains unsolved, precisely how, by what mechanism or mechanisms they achieve not only this catalogue of bad things, but also the presumed good they are credited with, i.e., reducing the incidence of these previously common diseases of childhood, and producing recognizable titers of specific antibodies against them in the blood of recipients.

In the case of the other vaccines at least, some of these answers are closer to being known, because they need various adjuvants and other toxic chemicals to accomplish their work, such as aluminum salts, thimerosal, formaldehyde, 2-phenoxyethanol, squalene, et al., which the investigation of adverse reactions has naturally focused upon. But the live viruses are capable of evoking a Th2 antibody response and a similar range of autoimmune diseases all by themselves, so to speak, without such chemicals. *How do they do it?* That is the question at the center of the whole business, and it still baffles my mind that nobody seems to be asking it.

Measles

As the most prevalent and typically the most intense of the three MMR diseases, measles has always attracted the most attention and been linked to the largest number and broadest array of complications. The most famous example of these was in the notorious 1998 *Lancet* paper of Andrew Wakefield and his colleagues, which demonstrated typical lesions of inflammatory bowel disease, as we saw, with specific antibodies against measles, but not mumps or rubella, in the intestinal lymphoid tissues of a number of autistic children.

But perhaps the most striking feature of the measles vaccine is that it was completely unnecessary. By the time I acquired the natural disease at the age of six, it had long since evolved from a killer disease into a normal disease of childhood, featuring an attack rate of close to 100%, which meant that almost everyone exposed to the virus came down with the disease, and almost everyone who did so not only recovered from it without complications or sequelae, but were also endowed as a result with the major lifelong benefits we have been discussing. After centuries of adaptation, together with improvements in sanitation and public health, the developed world, at least, had developed a relationship with the measles virus that was about as close to ideal as it could possibly be.

In short, the only plausible reason for mandating the vaccine must have been to showcase the effectiveness of the *concept*, by achieving its particular goal of drastically reducing the ubiquitous footprint of the disease. This it has most certainly done, and in spectacular fashion. But the mission of vaccinating everybody against it proved to be tragically shortsighted by throwing away the immense long-term benefits of coming down with and recovering from the acute disease, and contributing instead a substantial share of chronic, autoimmune diseases and deaths to the ongoing epidemic that continues unabated.

In retrospect, then, it has to be judged a tragic mistake, producing a counterfeit immunity that was never anything but partial, temporary, and incomplete, and achieving in the process an unhealthy reprogramming of the immune system that trades off the acute, vigorous responses to infection it was designed for in favor of weaker, but ongoing, chronic responses that have rendered us a lot sicker than we would have been had we simply left well enough alone.

As we saw, the small-scale measles outbreak of 2014 provided the CDC and the industry with a pretext to blame the parents of unvaccinated kids, and to agitate for eliminating their personal-belief exemptions,[38] rather than the vaccine itself, for its failure to protect the kids who *did* receive it. Just as has been shown with pertussis, children vaccinated with MMR also regularly shed live measles virus,[39] and could easily infect one another as well as the unvaccinated; the fact is that many outbreaks have taken place in populations where more than 95% of the cases have received the vaccine.[40]

Mumps and Rubella

The situation with mumps and rubella is similar, but with some distinctive variations. As with measles, outbreaks of mumps have continued; and the disease has similarly made a comeback in recent years, involving mainly adolescents and young adults of high school and college age, just as we would expect, in whom the partial, temporary immunity conferred by the vaccine has faded, and the risk of complications is considerably greater, mainly encephalitis, meningitis, deafness, orchitis, oophoritis, and infertility.[41]

Furthermore, when compared to the measles vaccine, the mumps component has been considerably less effective. Even though the average yearly incidence of the disease has plummeted by more than 99% since the vaccine was introduced,[42] large-scale outbreaks of several hundred to several thousand cases have continued to occur, which is especially remarkable since mumps is so much less contagious than measles, with an attack rate of only 30% or so.[43] In 2006, for example, there were a total of 6,584 cases, largely college students, scattered across 45 states, with a cluster of eight contiguous midwestern states accounting for 85% of them despite a mean two-dose vaccination coverage of 97%.[44] For actual cases of mumps whose vaccination status was known, the breakdown was unvaccinated, 12.7%; vaccinated with one dose, 24.8%.; and vaccinated with two doses, 62.5%.[45] In a similar 2009 outbreak involving 3,502 cases in New York and New Jersey, there were 2,317 cases with known vaccination status, of whom only 10% were unvaccinated, 14% had received one dose of vaccine, and 76% had received two doses.[46] In a recent outbreak at Harvard, there have been 41 cases so far, every one of them vaccinated.[47]

As for rubella, in school-age children the illness is usually so mild that it escapes detection; the vaccine was mandated in 1969 to prevent congenital rubella syndrome, which occurs mainly when rubella is contracted in the first trimester of pregnancy, and can result in miscarriage, fetal death, or a variety of birth defects. In adults, the main complication of rubella infection is arthritis, which can be severe. Since the disease has recently been declared "eliminated" from the United States and Latin America,[48] it is unnecessary to say anything more about it, except to question the truth of that boast, and to suggest that in any case there is no compelling reason to continue vaccinating against it.

SUMMARY

As the first three vaccines to be introduced after World War II, the DPT or DTaP, the IPV and OPV, and the MMR have all registered some degree of success in achieving their intended goals of reducing the prevalence of these diseases in their classic acute form, and of demonstrating specific antibodies in the serum of vaccinated individuals for extended periods of time.

But to a large extent these goals have proved illusory. In the first place, all of them have caused more than their share of serious adverse reactions, including death, various forms of brain damage, and a considerable array of autoimmune diseases, although the CDC and the industry have cleverly disqualified most of them from consideration, as we saw, by imposing arbitrarily rigid criteria that very few can satisfy. In the case of the DPT and DTaP, years of painstaking investigation have implicated its aluminum adjuvants in this same range of complications—notably autism and the various other forms of brain and nervous system impairment—that have become so shockingly prevalent since these vaccines were introduced.

For the MMR, the track record is similar, but includes a much wider array of autoimmune diseases as well as autism and brain damage, and without any conspicuous adjuvants to account for them. Clearly the live viruses can inflict the same kind and at least the same level of damage, but exactly how they do it remains mysterious.

Even more elusive in this respect are the polio vaccines, both OPV and IPV, which seemed much safer than the others, despite being prepared with the known toxins formaldehyde and 2-phenoxyethanol, until they were found to have been contaminated with the simian virus SV40 and to have produced many but still partly uncounted thousands of cancer cases that appeared only years later and are still being hotly contested by the vaccine establishment's well-oiled propaganda machine.

In the second place, their apparent success in reducing the incidence of these infections has been negated to a large extent by the CDC's redefinition of the disease, in case of paralytic polio, excluding all but the most serious and long-lasting cases, and by the emergence of vaccine-resistant strains through natural selection, even in some cases of related but completely different organisms, with the capacity to afflict human beings in much the same way. This evolution has been especially important in the case of pertussis, paralytic polio, and measles, the three most prominent diseases epidemiologically.

The most obvious example is pertussis, both of the vaccines against which were at best marginally effective to begin with, and have predictably engendered not only several resistant strains but a whole new species—*B. parapertussis*—resulting in a significant revival of a more virulent form of whooping cough in recent years, which had been dying off quite nicely on its own for many years before the vaccine was introduced.

Polio is unique not only in its exceedingly low attack rate, but also in having been covertly redefined to exclude all but the most serious chronic cases at precisely the same historical moment that the polio vaccine was first introduced, thus conveying the false impression that the vaccine had been responsible for the sudden drop in cases that quickly followed. In addition, in proportion to the decline in vaccine-strain polio cases, various countries have reported substantial increases in virtually identical clinical syndromes, such as non-polio acute flaccid paralysis (NPAFP) in India, and acute flaccid myelitis (AFM) in the United States, which latter has been traced to the related enterovirus D68.

Measles has so far resurfaced only in small-scale local outbreaks, and mumps in several larger ones; but the ineffectiveness of these vaccines in protecting vaccinated individuals during such outbreaks has so far had less to do with the emergence of resistant strains than with the inherent limitations of the vaccination concept, which applies to all vaccines, even and especially when they are successful in doing what they were intended to do.

As we saw, the most basic and important failing of vaccines is that they circumvent and indeed systematically weaken the normal immune response, the ensemble of coordinated mechanisms whereby infecting organisms are neutralized and expelled from the body. In lieu of that acute response to infection, vaccination substitutes the isolated technical feat of long-term antibody production, which evidently requires chronic, autoimmune reprogramming, so that even when no specific disease is present, we are diverted from achieving natural immunity, both specific and nonspecific, and the many profound health benefits that it confers.

Chapter 12

THE NEXT GENERATION

From the 1980s through the Clinton years, a whole new generation of single vaccines were introduced and mandated, namely, hepatitis B, Hib, pneumococcus, chicken pox, rotavirus, and influenza, along with some novel marketing strategies that deserve a closer look.

HEPATITIS B

The first of its kind, hepatitis B is a *recombinant* vaccine, meaning that its DNA has been genetically modified from that of the parent virus, a sleight-of-hand underlying the manufacturers' claim that it is no longer "alive," nor therefore capable of infecting anyone. So far, nobody has challenged them because technically viruses are "alive" only when they infect the cells of a living host.

But inasmuch as even the wild-type virus consists of nothing more than some DNA surrounded by a protein coat, and the latter is what supplies the antigens against which the vaccine is directed, the genetically modified version could still qualify as a virus, although nobody yet knows what illnesses might arise from it, let alone whether they happen to resemble hepatitis B or not. In short, the claim that it's not alive or infective amounts to a pious hope, if not a cynical word game. Since the bioengineered virus is only weakly antigenic, the vaccine also requires aluminum salts as adjuvants, and contains formaldehyde and yeast protein as well.[1]

As we saw, the hepatitis B vaccines are a test case of the industry's safety studies, which disqualify almost all autoimmune and chronic diseases from being considered vaccine-related simply because they often don't manifest or become diagnosable until weeks, months, or even years after the particular vaccine in question—well beyond the arbitrarily imposed narrow window of a few hours or days.

Hence, the glaring discrepancy between the official line of the industry and the CDC that the Hep B vaccine is among the safest now in use and the voluminous body of articles and case reports in the medical literature that link it not only to SIDS, autism, GBS, and the whole range of brain damage and neuropathology that we've come to expect from all vaccines adjuvanted with aluminum, but also to literally dozens of autoimmune diseases of every description, a dizzying array whose breadth and diversity are uniquely its own. Because at least some part of this morbidity has most likely arisen from the policy of giving the vaccine at birth, it is instructive to review how the Hep B mandate came about in the first place.

Comparatively widespread but seldom fatal, the disease known as hepatitis B can present itself acutely, chronically, or both. When chronic, it can multiply silently for many years and eventually lead to cirrhosis and permanent liver damage, which adds a further risk of liver cancer and death. Transmitted primarily through blood and to a lesser extent by sexual contact, the disease has long been a source of ill health among IV drug users, who still constitute its principal reservoir.

In the 1980s, the medical system belatedly took notice when hepatitis B and C, AIDS, and other blood-borne diseases began to appear as contaminants in donated blood, and thus to infect the medical and surgical patients in need of it, a looming scandal that pressured the blood banks to develop and implement more rigorous screening procedures.

When targeted vaccination campaigns consistently failed to reach the notoriously secretive drug subculture, the Hep B was mandated for everyone in 1991 as a last-ditch attempt to exert some degree of leverage over this seemingly intractable problem. Like a desperate "Hail-Mary" pass in the final seconds of a football game, the improbable strategy actually adopted was to vaccinate all newborn babies in the hospital so that those who later became drug addicts in their teens and twenties would at least be somewhat less likely to acquire the virus, and the blood supply would be protected to that extent. Sound far-fetched? Many pediatricians thought so at the time:

> "I don't see what the rush is," said one pediatrician at a UCSF conference, and neither did his audience. Only about a third of the 400 attendees said they were giving the vaccine routinely to infants. "We're trying to prevent a disease 25–30 years from now," he added. Others felt that children receive too many vaccines in the first year, and that each one is a disagreeable experience that may adversely affect compliance.[2]

Before long, the medical journals were inundated with letters of protest, many of them dubious that the vaccine would last long enough to do any good, and predicting that additional boosters would be needed later: "The patient handout falsely assures parents that the protective effects will last throughout the child's life, while the article admits that antibody levels decline over time, and booster shots may be needed. Since adolescents run the greatest risk of exposure, immunizing them might be more effective, and compliance would be higher."[3]

Nevertheless, most pediatricians were strongly committed to the vaccination concept as a general strategy for fighting infectious diseases, as indeed they still remain. By the mid-1990s the majority were actively on board with the campaign against Hep B just as reports of adverse autoimmune reactions began to be reported in large numbers, and it became their task to launder and sanitize them. Nevertheless, their original reservations about it have long since come true, but the wild impracticality of vaccinating all newborns against a disease of drug addicts that almost none of them will ever see has sadly been forgotten.

What should have dissuaded them was the unwisdom of vaccinating all newborn babies as their very first immunological experience—in effect a baptismal initiation into the religion of modern medicine—carried out with a bundle of spliced genetic material, aluminum salts, and a handful of foreign-protein antigens, a full-course menu for autoimmune phenomena, of a type and a level of pathological intensity to be determined by each in his own way, truly a "shot in the dark" of limitless possibility.

HAEMOPHILUS INFLUENZAE B

Hib is a *conjugate* vaccine, meaning that it attaches the capsular polysaccharide of the targeted *H. influenzae* bacterium, a weak antigen, to a much more strongly antigenic protein, in this case tetanus toxoid, so that the antibody response of the recipient, while prompted mainly by the toxoid, will also attack the polysaccharide, its intended target. With no adjuvants or live viruses to worry about, formaldehyde the only known toxin, and casein and beef heart infusion the only other foreign proteins in the mix,[4] we might expect a somewhat lower risk profile for the Hib than the DTaP, MMR, or Hep B; and indeed that prediction was seemingly borne out until fairly recently, when anecdotal case reports of type 1 diabetes, Guillain-Barré syndrome, transverse myelitis, and autoimmune thrombocytopenia began appearing, although deemed "insufficient to establish or reject a causal relationship" by the Institute of Medicine.[5] Since then, however, further evidence has since emerged to challenge those judgments, as we saw.[6]

Over and above the damage it has directly caused, another big problem with the Hib vaccine is the rationale for giving it in the first place, and what it says about the process by which vaccines are chosen for routine use, let alone mandated for all children. *Haemophilus influenzae* b, the bacterium targeted by the vaccine, is a mutant strain of the normal flora of the nasopharynx; and the Hib vaccine is the first that seeks to alter or interfere with this intricate microbiome, the product of uncounted generations of adaptive evolution.

Unquestionably, like many other such species, it can at times be a factor in both mild and serious diseases. It is one of the species most often cultured from the middle-ear fluid of infants and children with acute otitis media;[7] and has also played a role in bacterial meningitis, especially in young children under 5, and in pneumonia, epiglottitis, and pericarditis as well.

But in view of the fact that it lives peacefully among us most of the time, and undoubtedly keeps out many more uniformly hostile foreign organisms as well, it seems shortsighted and unwise to call it the *cause* rather than the *effect* of these illnesses, which presuppose some as yet unspecified alteration in the biochemistry of the blood and the nasopharyngeal environment that permits this usually tame organism to revert to wildness and multiply without restraint. Nobody would disagree that people seriously ill with potentially life-threatening diseases need help to recover, but it surely makes better sense to take care of our normal flora by maintaining an optimal environment for them to live in harmony than to attack and kill them in everyone, as we would an enemy, to prevent illnesses that the vast majority of us will never experience.

All of which brings me to wonder, as I often do, who gets to decide that diseases like Hib or hepatitis B have become such imminent and serious threats to the public health that the entire population must be vaccinated against them, with or without their consent? It is not difficult to conjure up a pretty close approximation of what actually happens in real life: a conference room in Washington, where representatives of the CDC, the FDA, the American Academy of Pediatrics, the ACIP, and the manufacturers themselves put their heads together to decide which vaccines to promote or mandate next, and what marketing strategy to devise for them. But the most important feature of these deliberations is that you and I and the general public have absolutely no part in them.

In the short term, the vaccine does appear to have been moderately successful in reducing the incidence of invasive Hib diseases, especially meningitis and otitis media;[8] and the predicted serotype replacement has not yet become a serious problem, at least in school-age children, according to many different sources.[9] But a 2003 study from Brazil showed that *H. influenzae* meningitis type a, hitherto of minor importance, had already increased eightfold within a year of beginning the vaccination program,[10] an ominous development for the future.

THE PNEUMOCOCCUS

Resembling the Hib in many ways, the pneumococcus vaccines are also conjugates, employing a protein antigen derived from diphtheria toxin (but not the toxoid), and a structurally similar capsular polysaccharide that is likewise equated with virulence. It does, however, contain an aluminum adjuvant, which two of the three Hib vaccines do not, as well as the detergent polysorbate 80.[11] Like the Hib, the pneumococcus organism is an important component of the normal flora of the nasopharynx; and at times when that microhabitat becomes altered in ways not yet well understood, it has similarly been implicated in a comparable spectrum of invasive diseases, chiefly, otitis media, sinusitis, meningitis, pneumonia, sepsis, and endocarditis.

In the 1970s, long before the Hib vaccine made its appearance, the first pneumococcal version was introduced in an attempt to prevent bacterial pneumonia in the elderly, especially in overcrowded nursing homes and residential facilities, where pneumococci were the species most frequently identified. But it proved ineffective in this already debilitated population, as in this study of ambulatory but high-risk, middle-aged and elderly patients in the VA system:

> We conducted a randomized, double-blind, placebo-controlled trial to test the efficacy of a pneumococcal polysaccharide vaccine in 2,295 high-risk patients with one or more of the following: age 55+, diabetes, alcoholism, chronic cardiac, pulmonary, hepatic, or renal disease. We were unable to prove any efficacy of the vaccine in preventing either pneumonia or bronchitis in this population.[12]

In the wake of such studies, the vaccine never attained broad popularity with either the target population or their doctors, who continued to use it without enthusiasm until the Clinton years, when the war on childhood ear infections was intensifying and the time-honored strategy of aggressive antibiotic treatment was exposed as a dismal failure.[13]

In the late 1990s, the vaccine was duly recycled for pediatric use when it was found to be somewhat effective in preventing acute otitis media, in which the pneumococcus likewise plays a major role.[14] Here at last was the marketing strategy that the CDC and the industry had been waiting for; they have promoted the vaccine aggressively ever since, not only for young children, but also increasingly for adolescents, young adults, mature adults, and even middle-aged fifty-somethings of the AARP set,[15] as if it might soon qualify as a panacea for the entire population and need to be repeated throughout life.

Yet a sizable number of pediatricians have continued to resist this vaccine, and also, at least implicitly, its underlying strategy of recklessly altering our resident flora without knowing or even caring about the long-term consequences. In 2001, for example, after the Finnish Otitis Media Study reported that the new vaccine was effective in preventing ear infections, several readers were quick to cite the serotype replacement that was already taking place:

> The manufacturer concludes that the new vaccine is effective for prevention. But the data do not support this conclusion. As the authors admit, the treated group could have had more episodes than the controls. In 1999, these same data were presented to the FDA, which rejected using this vaccine in otitis media. But the most interesting results are ecological. In a short time the predicted serotype replacement observed with other bacterial vaccines was realized. With this clear warning sign, it is ecologically perilous to push this vaccine.[16]

An even more telling criticism came from a pediatrician in the Netherlands, where ear infections are common but rarely medicated or even considered a major public health issue:

> According to the protocol, all infants received four vaccinations, which prevented only 6% of cases. More could be gained by changing our *attitude* toward acute otitis media, which in the Netherlands is seen as a self-limiting disease. Often parents do not take their children to the doctor for it, and antibiotics are only moderately effective anyway. As has been shown, educating parents and doctors will lead to a decrease in antibiotic prescriptions.[17]

Characteristically, the industry has tackled the problem of serotype replacement by simply including more and more serotypes in the vaccine, with Wyeth graduating from its heptavalent Prevnar-7 to the 13-valent Prevnar-13, and Merck coming in with its own version, Pneumovax-23. But with a whole generation of bacteria turning over within a few hours, it requires no rocket science to anticipate that the natural evolutionary process will quickly outsmart these blundering attempts to manipulate and control it, a process already well under way.

CHICKEN POX

Like the MMR, with which it is often combined, the varicella is a live-virus vaccine. While needing no adjuvants, disinfectants, or preservatives, it does contain the antibiotic neomycin, the chelating agent ethylenediamine tetra-acetic acid (EDTA), the excitatory neurotransmitter glutamate, and above all, a considerable assortment of foreign cells and proteins, like human embryonic lung cell cultures, WI-38 human diploid cell cultures (fibroblasts from a female fetus that was aborted in 1964), MRC-5 human diploid cell cultures (from a 14-week male fetus that was aborted in 1966), bovine fetal and calf serum, and embryonic guinea pig cell cultures.[18]

The Merck vaccine dates from the 1960s; but like the pneumococcus, it was never used on a large scale until the Clinton years, when government enthusiasm for all vaccination programs attained such dizzying heights that a plausible rationale could at last be invented for marketing it. Even then, it was not an easy sell, since chicken pox is an illness so innocuous that the *AMA Encyclopedia of Medicine* described it as "a common, mild infectious disease, to which all healthy children should be exposed at an age when it is no more than an inconvenience."[19] As late as 1996, even the American Academy of Pediatrics, which yields to no one in its righteous and fanatical zeal for vaccinations of every kind, echoed this traditional view in its patient brochure, based on the pooled clinical experience of many generations of physicians everywhere:

> Most children who get chicken pox and are otherwise healthy experience no complications from it. When adults get it, the disease usually lasts longer and is more severe, often developing into pneumonia. Adults are almost 10 times more likely than children under fourteen to need hospitalization for the disease and more than 20 times more likely to die from it.[20]

After decades of failed attempts, for Merck to have been able to persuade competitors and government regulators alike to welcome a vaccine against a disease that was so common and so easily overcome—not to mention securing a universal mandate for it, including exclusive "sweetheart" deals with federal and state agencies that guaranteed millions of doses at their chosen price—has to be reckoned among the most spectacular coups in modern corporate history and immediately raises the question of how they pulled it off.

Although the CDC's Information Statement still tells parents that its main purpose is to prevent the serious complications listed, saving 100 deaths annually would hardly qualify as a public health emergency, were it not for the fervent, quasi-religious belief in vaccination as an automatic "win-win" across the board; but Merck had already been playing that card for decades without success.

All that had changed was the new financial argument making the rounds among Clinton administration officials, that universal vaccination of children was generating huge savings in social costs for the *parents,* chiefly in lost wages and extra day care, a novel approach that quickly made its way into this brochure from the American Academy of Family Physicians, which was handed out to parents as their kids were offered up:

> **Why is a vaccine needed?** Chicken pox is usually a mild illness, but can cause problems like brain swelling, pneumonia, and skin infections. It may be very serious in infants and adults. Because it is so contagious, children shouldn't go to school or day care until all the sores have dried or crusted. Many parents miss work during the illness, because of which the lost pay can be a significant cost to them.[21]

What is particularly revealing about this little document is its implied subtext, namely,

1. Even though the disease is so mild, the children still need to be protected from it.
2. Even when vaccinated, they still need to be isolated from their friends and classmates, even if they too have been vaccinated.

Purely from the viewpoint of logic and common sense, what this all amounts to is that the vaccine doesn't protect any given individual very effectively, which is unfortunately true. Furthermore, even though the economic argument turns out to be false, as I will presently show, it does reflect a significant change in society, that few children today enjoy the good fortune and indeed the luxury of a stay-at-home parent to nurse them through the chicken pox, measles, or whatever, as I and so many of my contemporaries did two generations ago, so that the now-standard, two-paycheck family must indeed often incur a loss of income when the children get sick and have to stay home.

In any case, just as with the Hep B and pneumococcus, many physicians were lukewarm to the chicken pox program in the beginning, most expressing the worries that had already materialized in the case of the MMR, chiefly, the inevitable waning of immunity in adolescents and young adults associated with more severe illness and a much higher risk of complications, as was well-known:

> Chicken pox has long been a benign disease of preschool- and school-aged children. Although immunization is supposedly axiomatic for public health, vaccinating all kids against chicken pox is a bad idea. It is unknown whether long-term immunity arises from an attack of the disease, or from the virus repeatedly boosting it in our communities, or how long immunity will last after the shot. Over time, mass vaccination will eradicate most naturally occurring varicella and its booster effect. If the immunity of vaccinated kids wanes with age, and unvaccinated kids escape disease because contagion is rarer, life-threatening outbreaks may occur as these kids grow older. Since morbidity and mortality are increased in fetuses and after childhood, an ever-expanding population with unboosted or waning immunity, including pregnant women, may be created.[22]

But once again, these various doubts, quibbles, and qualifications, well-intentioned and prophetic though they proved to be, were quickly drowned out by a carefully orchestrated program of blustering and bullying from the vaccine establishment, exemplified by this *JAMA* editorial from two Yale pediatricians that concluded with the following peroration:

> Do the benefits of universal immunization outweigh the risks? Many studies show the risk of complications from *Varicella* in normal children, and there is evidence that they have been underestimated. Others show that the vaccine is cost-effective. Why would we deny children protection from this unpleasant rite of passage when the evidence is so favorable? Time to stop procrastinating, and JUST DO IT![23]

In any case, just like the Hep B, Hib, and pneumococcus, the chicken pox has long since become routine, and is mostly given without question or demur, although a fair number of parents still refuse it and even try to expose their kids when sporadic cases appear. Nor can it be doubted that it has "worked," since the incidence of the disease, which in the early 1990s accounted for an average of about 150,000 cases annually in the US,[24] has plummeted by 85% since the mandate, and the serious cases by 95%.[25]

But these nominal successes look a lot less impressive when set against the equally marked increases in shingles,[26] beginning in progressively younger age groups and with considerably more pain and suffering, not to mention more numerous and costly drugs and doctor visits. In addition, it has already been linked at least provisionally to a considerable array of autoimmune diseases that are listed in the package insert, namely, encephalitis and encephalopathy, Guillain-Barré syndrome, transverse myelitis, Bell's palsy, stroke, ataxia, seizures, Stevens-Johnson syndrome, thrombocytopenic purpura, aplastic anemia, angio-edema, Henoch-Schönlein purpura, and erythema multiforme,[27] with I daresay plenty more to come.

But perhaps worst of all, and certainly the most difficult to quantify, are the diseases that would have been prevented or at least restrained by not vaccinating, as we saw,[28] namely, various forms of cancer (ear, nose, and throat, ovarian, genital, prostate, GI tract, lung, brain, and melanoma), inflammatory bowel disease (Crohn's, ulcerative colitis), type 1 diabetes (IDDM), asthma, allergies, and coronary disease; at least, these are the ones that have been documented thus far. Far from saving money, I'd call it penny-wise and pound-foolish.

ROTAVIRUS

Another live-virus vaccine, like the chicken pox, the two rotavirus offerings are administered orally, and are likewise free of adjuvants, disinfectants, and preservatives; but they do contain antibiotics (neomycin, chlortetracycline, and amphotericin-B), the detergent polysorbate 80, the chelating agent EDTA, the neurotransmitter glutamate, and the usual quota of foreign cells and proteins, namely, chicken fibroblasts, human serum albumin, bovine serum, chicken proteins, and bovine gelatin.[29]

Like the chicken pox, rotavirus vaccines appeared on the scene in the late 1990s, backed by a similar cost-benefit analysis, and should be kept under glass in a museum as a specimen of the peculiar mentality that led to it, and a cautionary tale about what we should expect even more of in the future.

In the pre-vaccine era, according to the CDC's Rotavirus Information Statement, there were an average of 400,000 doctor visits annually for the disease, as well as 200,000 trips to the ER, 60,000 hospitalizations, and 40 deaths; and since the vaccine, all of these figures have indeed fallen considerably.[30] In 1996, the *Journal of the AMA* published a CDC report that advocated mass vaccination against it:

> Rotavirus is the most common cause of severe diarrhea among young children in the US. Although it causes few deaths in this country, it causes 50,000 hospitalizations and $550,000,000 in direct medical costs annually. Safe live oral vaccines have been developed that will prevent 50–60% of the diarrhea and 70–100% of the severest cases. The decision to implement a national vaccination program will be based on the expected reduction in severe outcomes and cost-effectiveness. A previous study found that it would yield net savings of $80,000,000 in health-care costs and $465,000,000 in social costs, based on the price of $20 per dose.[31]

By their own math, however, the authors calculated a saving of only $300 million in social costs, and a net *increase* of $100 million in health-care costs, which could only be offset by lowering the price of the vaccine to the break-even point of $9 per dose.[32] Tackling the same issue, an editorial in the *New England Journal of Medicine* pointed out that the vaccine would be extremely effective in the developing world, where rotavirus and other infectious diarrheas pose an enormous public health problem and are a major cause of death, but would be affordable and profitable only in affluent countries like our own:

> Diarrhea is no longer a serious threat in the United States. It remains common, but its severity has diminished to about 300 deaths per year. On the other hand, the vaccine is safe and can prevent nearly half of the cases, 80% of the severe ones, and nearly all of the dehydration. An effective program would significantly reduce mortality, hospitalization, and other medical costs, estimated at $500–600 million annually, as well as the indirect costs, including lost wages and the cost of child care. When is too much too much? *One hundred preventable deaths are too many, and $500,000,000 in direct health-care costs is too high.* Hence a safe and effective vaccine, even at $30 per dose, can be recommended for routine use in the US and developed countries.[33]

What is really striking about this argument is not just what we already know, that these Clinton-era mandates are publicly justified as a way of saving money, rather than any imminent or large-scale threat to the public health, but also that their ultimate motive is a fanatical ambition to root out disease wherever it appears, no matter what the cost, and even—as in this case—to the extent of being useless and quite possibly dangerous by its own calculation.

Although doubtless understated by an unknown but considerable factor, suppose that we accept the CDC's figures for the moment, and even their moral calculus that saving 100 kids' lives from rotavirus disease or the chicken pox is sufficient cause to inject tens of millions of kids with these vaccines every year. Suppose further that our vaccination campaign is hugely successful, that we inject, say, 25 million kids with rotavirus every year; that the incidence of the disease drops precipitously; and that the CDC's lowball estimate of 1 in 20,000 reports of intussusception is accurate. That still adds up to at least 1,250 life-threatening cases of intestinal obstruction per year. If we then remember the CDC's admission that these reports constitute only 10% of the real total, we get a somewhat more realistic although still probably undercounted total of 12,500 life-threatening obstructions annually.

In other words, to save those 100 lives, we have to risk the lives of at least 12,500, most of whom will require surgery if their cases are discovered in time, and some of whom will very likely die or suffer permanent and crippling injury, not to mention injecting 25 million healthy kids with a virus that they may never encounter and would almost invariably recover from if they did. Like the "War on Terror," this amounts to a quasi-religious crusade, a declaration of endless war on disease, indeed the polar opposite of a prudent, sensible, and well-reasoned public health strategy.

Nor are these cases of intussusception by any means the whole story. We haven't yet factored in the toll of autoimmune diseases that have been automatically disqualified from consideration, as we saw,[34] especially those that take more time to develop than allowed under the tidy little guidelines that the CDC and the industry have devised for that purpose. As it turns out, while designed to prevent an illness that is almost always mild and nonthreatening, the rotavirus vaccines have already been linked to urticaria, angionedema, and Kawasaki disease, an autoimmune vasculitis that causes inflammation of medium-sized arteries anywhere in the body with high fever, and can be fatal if untreated. It requires no crystal ball or gift of prophecy to anticipate that more than a few others will be added to the list in the years to come.

In 1998, the first rotavirus vaccine, Rotashield, developed by Wyeth-Lederle, was recommended for all infants, even though five cases of intussusception had already been reported in the test population for a risk of 0.5%.[35] In the first eight months of the program, many new cases were discovered; the vaccine was quietly withdrawn pending further investigation, which confirmed "a causal association" between the vaccine and intussusception" that was "strong, temporal, and specific," and much more prevalent than the original trials had indicated.[36] In 1999, the ACIP withdrew its recommendation, the vaccine was hastily recalled, and the whole affair was hushed up as if nothing had happened.

In 2006, two new live rotavirus vaccines were introduced, which have so far avoided scandal, but they still list intussusception as a side effect in the package insert along with the other complications previously discussed. But even without any comparably scandalous revelations in the future, it is the *concept* of the vaccine with its two opposite and indeed incompatible rationales that fails to measure up to any legitimate, practical need or genuine public health imperative.

In view of the above, it should occasion no surprise that RotaTeq, Merck's rotavirus offering, has already netted a considerable fortune for Dr. Paul Offit, who owns the patent, and who, as you may recall, once famously said that a human infant can easily tolerate 10,000 vaccines simultaneously,[37] while serving on the ACIP at the moment it came up for approval and for many years thereafter.[38]

INFLUENZA

But I've saved the best for last; in several respects, the influenza vaccine tops them all. Here are some choice excerpts from the CDC's Vaccine Information Statement:

> **Why get vaccinated?**
> Influenza ("flu") is a contagious disease that spreads around the United States every year, usually between October and May. Flu is caused by influenza viruses, and is spread mainly by coughing, sneezing, and close contact. Anyone can get flu. It strikes suddenly and can last several days. Symptoms vary, but can include fever and chills, sore throat, muscle aches, fatigue, cough, headache, and runny or stuffy nose. It can also lead to pneumonia and blood infections, and cause diarrhea and seizures in children. If you have a medical condition, such as heart or lung disease, flu can make it worse. It is also more dangerous for infants and young children, people over 65 years, pregnant women, and those with certain health conditions or a weakened immune system.
>
> Each year thousands of people in the United States die from flu, and many more are hospitalized. Flu vaccine can keep you from getting flu, make flu less severe if you do get it, and keep you from spreading it to your family and others.
>
> A dose of flu vaccine is recommended every flu season. Children from six months through eight years of age may need two doses during the same flu season. Everyone else needs only one dose each flu season.

Some inactivated flu vaccines contain a very small amount of a mercury-based preservative called Thimerosal. Studies have not shown it to be harmful in vaccines, but flu vaccines that do not contain it are available.

There is no live flu virus in flu shots; they cannot cause the flu. There are many flu viruses, and they are always changing. Each year a new flu vaccine is made to protect against three or four viruses that are likely to cause disease in the upcoming flu season. But even when the vaccine doesn't exactly match these viruses, it may still provide some protection.

Flu vaccine cannot prevent flu that is caused by a virus not covered by the vaccine, or illnesses that look like flu but are not.

Risks

Minor problems: localized soreness, redness, swelling; sore, red, itchy eyes; hoarseness, cough, fever; headache, aches, and fatigue.

Serious problems: a small increased risk of Guillain-Barré Syndrome, 1–2 cases per 1,000,000 doses.[39]

•

Although free of adjuvants, the flu vaccine contains formaldehyde, the detergents polysorbate-80, octoxynol-10, and sodium deoxycholate, the antibiotic gentamicin sulfate, hydrocortisone, embryonated chicken eggs, and egg albumin; the multi-dose vials still contain thimerosal as well.[40]

We have already surveyed the most serious adverse effects of vaccines, namely, a broad spectrum of autoimmune diseases and brain damage, sometimes leading to death, in substantial numbers of susceptible individuals. On the other hand, as we have seen, some of them have at least accomplished their intended goals of reducing the morbidity and mortality of the diseases that correspond to them.

But the influenza vaccine, notwithstanding repeated mass campaigns of unprecedented scope, cannot boast of having achieved any comparable success whatsoever, in part because of two built-in disadvantages that are clearly and prominently stated in the CDC's own Information Statement. The manufacturers could have saved themselves a lot of time and money, and the public a significant toll of death and serious injury, if they had simply paid attention to what they already knew, and directed their energies to more genuinely pressing issues.

The first problem is that influenza viruses are highly unstable genetically, with a known propensity for mutating from season to season, and even from week to week sometimes, such that the vaccine has to be redesigned every year, yet must also be based to some extent on the previous year's version plus a considerable dose of guesswork, with the virtually inevitable result of very limited and sometimes no measurable effect at all on the new strain or strains. Yet the industry and its physician-advocates have cannily morphed this very unpredictability into an argument for giving the shot every year, and thus exponentially multiplied both the margin of profit and the risk of loss, from the millions of doses that their contracted health departments and agencies might agree or sometimes decline to buy at the last minute.

The second problem is that many cases of the illness we all know as "the flu," with its characteristic picture of fever and chills, nonspecific aches and pains, profound fatigue and muscular weakness, and assorted upper-respiratory or digestive disturbances, or both, is also caused by many viruses other than the influenza group for which it is named. In practice, clinicians often simply write it off as "the flu," just as patients do, without knowing or caring whether the virus is actually present, or without going to the trouble of finding out.

For both reasons, it can hardly be a surprise that influenza vaccines have consistently failed to show any significant benefit, and indeed would almost surely fail even if they were entirely successful in preventing infections by the particular strains they happen to be directed against.

Technically, the influenza vaccine doesn't even belong in this chapter, since it was first given to the military in World War II and marketed for general use in the late 1940s, making it even older than the MMR or polio.[41] After what seemed a promising start, careful analysis of the first major postwar outbreak in 1947 showed the incidence of disease to have been essentially the same in those who were vaccinated and those who were not;[42] but the vaccine was approved for general use nevertheless. Similarly, during the "Asian flu" pandemic of 1957–58, which caused about 2 million deaths worldwide and prompted the development of a new vaccine, it too was an abysmal failure, although there were far fewer US cases than its proponents had warned of,[43] another pattern that has often dogged its history.

In both instances, and indeed ever since, the official excuse has always been inadequate coverage. In 1960, routine annual vaccination was recommended for everyone, especially the elderly and chronically ill, a policy widely adopted by the early 1960s, ignoring a 1964 study by the CDC itself that found no convincing evidence for its having succeeded, and no compelling reason for continuing it.[44] In 1968, the CDC commissioned another randomized, double-blind trial of the current flu vaccine, and again found that it had no significant effect on morbidity or mortality.[45]

In 1976, detection of the H1N1 or so-called "swine flu" strain, similar to that of the global pandemic of 1918, predictably gave rise to yet another massive vaccination campaign, with essentially the same result as before, no consistent effect on morbidity and mortality, and further complicated by the fact that the H1N1 strain largely failed to materialize in the predicted numbers, yet hundreds of cases of Guillain-Barré syndrome kept popping up in its wake, giving rise to an unprecedented volume of litigation and hefty damage awards from the manufacturers.[46] Once again, the CDC was forced to concede that the vaccine had been ineffective.[47]

Much the same pattern has prevailed ever since, with repeated studies showing each new incarnation of the vaccine to be ineffective in reducing morbidity and mortality, yet being consistently drowned out by the repeated drumbeat of the manufacturers and government agencies alike that they are safe and effective. What is different, and what persuaded me to include the vaccine in this chapter, is that, roughly coinciding with the 1986 law establishing the Vaccine Court, and the defunding of public health agencies by the "free-market" conservatives who have dominated Congress ever since, the CDC and the medical establishment have evolved into something more or less indistinguishable from the mouthpiece for the industry, as we saw.[48]

As with the other vaccines discussed in this chapter, and also the MMR which preceded them, the influenza perfectly summarizes the extraordinary expansion of the vaccination concept, which was inspired originally by the threat of life-threatening epidemic diseases like smallpox, into a virtual talisman or panacea against infectious diseases of every description, simply because we have the technical capacity to make them, largely without restraint or regulation, and essentially as a spur to scientific innovation for its own sake, in the name of which certain sacrifices will inevitably and unfortunately have to be made.

Once again, beginning in the Clinton years and uninterruptedly ever since, the history of the flu vaccine has been one of newsworthy defeats cleverly repackaged as cutting-edge victories. Thus in 1995, an FDA review warned of too little randomization and other serious design flaws in existing safety and efficacy trials,[49] while in 2000 even the CDC reluctantly admitted that on the whole the flu vaccine had failed on economic grounds,[50] which had become the main argument in its favor.

Nevertheless, in 2004 the American Academy of Pediatrics recommended the annual flu shot not only for young children, but also for their household contacts; in many places it became mandatory for nurses and other health-care providers,[51] more than a few of whom were fired for refusing it.[52] Still other studies were commissioned to proclaim its worth for healthy young adults in the workforce,[53] and most improbably of all for pregnant women, exempted as inviolable until then, on the flimsy ground of protecting their newborns from the risk of RSV and bronchiolitis, even though these conditions involve a different group of viruses altogether.[54]

In any case, quite apart from these much-heralded successes and privately admitted failures, the real bottom line for the flu vaccine is the number of its victims, whose deaths, disabling injuries, and serious diseases are similar in kind, but if anything even greater in magnitude to those we are already familiar with. While the Vaccine Information Statement makes it sound like one of the safest available, it is by far the leading cause of damage awards by the Vaccine Court, even though these represent but a tiny fraction of the real total, as we saw.

In the fourth quarter of 2013, for example, the VICP compensated 75 people for their injuries, of which 42, or 56%, were from the flu vaccine; they encompassed a wide range of neurological injuries, including vertigo, peripheral neuropathy, cerebellar ataxia, myoclonus, blindness, optic neuritis, multiple sclerosis, leukoencephalopathy, transverse myelitis, chronic inflammatory demyelinating polyneuropathy, and Guillain-Barré syndrome, which last accounted for 24 cases, more than the rest of them put together, as well as other non-neurological complaints, such as chronic fatigue syndrome (CFS), fibromyalgia, myopathy, myositis, muscle wasting, chronic pain and muscle weakness, and death.[55]

For purposes of comparison, here are the damage awards for other vaccines during the same period, showing very much the same spread, and the typical aggravation from giving multiple vaccines simultaneously:

DTaP and IPV	encephalopathy
DT	SIRVA (vaccine-related shoulder injury)
Tdap, Hep B, and MMR	GBS, severe cognitive & emotional sequelae
Td	GBS
Tetanus	demyelinating injury
DTaP & Meningococcus	transverse myelitis
Tetanus	GBS
HPV	acute demyelinating encephalomyelitis
Hep B	orthostatic hypotension
DTaP	recurrent cluster headaches
DTaP, Hib, and MMR	juvenile dermatomyositis
DTaP, IPV, Hep B, Hib, Pneumo,	encephalopathy, death

HPV	multiple sclerosis
Pneumo, Varicella, and MMR	encephalopathy
Td	severe CFS, chronic pain, muscle weakness
DTaP and Hib	myoclonus
Tdap and Hep B	SIRVA, rheumatoid arthritis
Tdap	paresthesia, joint pains, and weakness
Meningococcus	vasculitis, disfiguring
Tetanus and Hep B	seizures, shoulder and neck pain, myositis, radiculopathy, severe neuropathies
Tdap	weakness, fatigue, headaches, paresthesia
Hep B, Hib, IPV, DTaP, Pneumo	death
Tdap	brachial neuritis
DTaP, MMR	thrombocytopenic purpura
HPV	polymyositis
Tetanus	transverse myelitis
Hep B	focal lipodystrophy with paresthesias[56]

Under "Fluarix" in the *Physicians' Desk Reference,* I found still more serious adverse reactions listed:

- tachycardia, vasculitis, lymphadenopathy, and Henoch-Schönlein purpura;
- angioedema, erythema multiforme, and Stevens-Johnson syndrome;
- chest pain and abdominal pain;
- abscess and cellulitis;
- anaphylaxis and serum sickness;
- tonsillitis, facial palsy, vertigo, and syncope;
- asthma, bronchospasm, and dyspnea.[57]

As we saw, everyone agrees that the adverse reactions reported to the VAERS system are far below the real figure, while the criteria for a reported injury to be considered as vaccine-related are designed to be all but impossible to satisfy.[58] But whether the real figure is 10 times greater, as the CDC estimates, or 100 times greater, as the former head of the FDA thought, or 1,000 times greater, as our experienced ER nurse passionately insisted, the truth is that we don't really know; and thanks to all of the obfuscations outlined above, we will probably never find out.

SUMMARY

In the generation following the introduction of "the Big Three," culminating in the 1990s, several new vaccines were developed, marketed, and eventually mandated for all children, namely, hepatitis B, Hib, pneumococcus, chicken pox, rotavirus, and influenza, an older vaccine that became mandatory during this period. The Hib and pneumococcus are directed against organisms of the normal flora, while the chicken pox and rotavirus are live viruses; the Hep B has been genetically engineered; and the influenza is in a category all by itself.

What they all have in common is that their corresponding natural diseases were and still are rarely fatal, and the vaccines were developed primarily to save the parental costs of lost wages and child care, or (in the case of Hep B) to reach the notoriously wary population of IV drug users, by vaccinating the captive audience of newborn babies in the hospital during the very first days of their extrauterine life.

In every case, even when their short-term goals were successfully attained, these strategies have ultimately backfired in at least three important respects. Although comparatively simple in design and seemingly a little less toxic than the others, the Hib and pneumococcus inevitably and predictably altered the natural balance of the resident nasopharyngeal bacteria, a delicate ecosystem of enormous importance for health, by promoting the emergence of resistant strains, as we saw with the pertussis and polio vaccines, and of modified versions of the target illness along with them.

Even more ominous than this immediate effect was the precedent it set, the entitlement and indeed the license, so far unchallenged, for continuing to manipulate our natural biome, the product of centuries and millennia of evolution, more or less at will, and without restraint, regulation, or any deep understanding of or even concern about the subtler energies at play, or their effect on our long-term health and well-being.

The live-virus vaccines, chicken pox and rotavirus, were likewise completely unnecessary because both illnesses are well-controlled, typically mild in children, and seldom fatal, at least in the developed world, and because coming down with and recovering from them confer many of the same important health benefits that we have seen for measles, mumps, rubella, and other acute, febrile illnesses of childhood. Moreover, as we've come to expect, they are far from innocuous, each with a significant array of diseases linked to it.

To begin with, the Hep B is an absurdly foolish idea, since it is given to babies to prevent a disease that few of them will ever see, and since those who do come down with it will do so only twenty years later or more. Secondly, it is also among the most dangerous of the vaccines, not only because of the aluminum it contains, with all the neuropathology that goes with it, but also because of the unparalleled diversity of autoimmune diseases that are linked to it, involving every tissue and organ system.

Third, by altering the virus's DNA, the manufacturers have opened a Pandora's box of still other possible diseases, both old and new, both known and unknown, that will be difficult if not impossible to close again. And fourth, it is given to all newborn babies as their very first immunological experience, when their blood-brain barrier is still largely unformed, and their brains and central nervous systems are thus exquisitely vulnerable to every form of serious and permanent damage.

As for the influenza vaccine, it has never worked, and *will* never work, because the virus is so mutable that any vaccine against it will be obsolete by the time it's ready for use, and because the illness we know as "the flu" is produced by many viruses, not merely the influenza group that gives it its name. Including several conducted by the CDC itself, study after study have shown it to be ineffective; but the industry and their physician-advocates have persuaded everyone to accept the flu shot every year, from the cradle to grave, and now in the womb as well, since even the pregnant woman, her fetus, and her newborn baby are to be protected against a virus that is smarter than the vaccine, and that virtually everyone recovers from anyway.

It thus encompasses all of the themes of this chapter, as the supreme example of why and how most vaccines don't work, and of how taking them not only imposes serious risks of injury and death, but also deprives recipients of the important and permanent health benefits of learning how to respond acutely and vigorously to infections, as our immune systems are clearly designed to do.

Chapter 13

PRESENT AND FUTURE

GENERAL TRENDS

Along with their development, the marketing and eventual mandating of new vaccines continue without letup, restraint, or effective regulation. The ACIP Schedule of Recommended Vaccines has recently added several more to the list, both for children and adults, with literally hundreds still in the pipeline, many beginning to be directed against cancer and other chronic diseases rather than infections, and several involving entirely new DNA technologies with ominous risks of their own, as I shall presently describe.

This major escalation of already existing trends also highlights an underlying motive of the industry and the medical system alike, which might even have served as an excuse for the suffering and death caused by vaccines were it not so implacably cruel—namely, the inexorable forward march of technology itself, fueled by all-too-human greed and ambition, as we have seen.

Although developing safer vaccines would require nothing more elaborate than identifying those at highest risk for adverse reactions, and broadening the personal-belief exemption, the industry and its allies in medicine, politics, and science have thus far paid scant attention to such pleas. But their time may be running out: slowly and incrementally, the sheer number and extent of vaccine programs seem to be undermining the widespread public acceptance that their prodigious commercial success was built upon.

MENINGOCOCCUS

Causally linked to the bacterium *Neisseria meningitidis*, a relative of the organism responsible for gonorrhea, meningococcal disease takes the form of meningitis and often an associated septicemia or blood infection, both of which can be rapidly fatal and carry a high risk of residual brain damage and other sequelae. Even with proper treatment, the death rate can reach 10%, and that of long-term disability almost 20%.[1]

On the other hand, the disease is uncommon, and has become increasingly so; the CDC reported an annual total of roughly 3,500–4,500 cases from 1970 to 2000, and a rapid decline since then, totaling only 550 cases in 2013.[2] Furthermore, along with other *Neisseria* species, the organism *N. meningitidis* is a common inhabitant of the nasopharyngeal flora, especially in a sizable minority of adolescents and adults, roughly 20% of whom harbor it without any illness whatsoever;[3] so once again, as with the Hib and pneumococcus, we must question the wisdom of sacrificing however many children to our overweening desire to find out exactly what will happen without any clear public health imperative for doing so.

Like the Hib and pneumococcus, the various meningococcal vaccines are conjugates, in which the organism's capsular polysaccharide is attached to tetanus toxoid or diphtheria toxoid to enhance its antigenicity; and much the same kind of serotype conversion can be expected to occur as well. Originally, it was developed primarily to avert small outbreaks of meningitis among adolescents and young adults in high schools, colleges, universities, and other crowded situations, where the disease is most likely to occur and spread; the newest versions have been modified to be suitable for infants as well. It has been recommended for adolescents since 2005, and as of 2016 it is mandated in 28 states.[4]

In addition, the older vaccines contain the following ingredients that are either known to be toxic or suspected of being so, namely, thimerosal (in Menoimmune, the Sanofi-Pasteur version), formaldehyde, beef extract, yeast extract, casein, and beef heart.[5] The two newest vaccines, Bexsero and Trumenba, are directed against the B strain, which the earlier versions did not address, and are conjugated with recombinant (i.e., bioengineered) proteins derived from the bacterium *E. coli*, the main inhabitant of our intestinal flora, yet another shot in the dark into our perilous future.[6]

Addressing the University of Colorado student government's proposed mandate for all incoming students, Robert F. Kennedy Jr. has shown, based on the CDC's own figures, that the risk of dying from the vaccine far exceeds that of dying from the disease, and possibly even of contracting it, as Gordon Stewart realized for the pertussis vaccine long ago:

> According to their package inserts, the older vaccines produce "serious adverse events" in 1% of recipients. If you inoculate Colorado's 400,000 college students

with them, you can expect 4,000 serious adverse events and 12 deaths. We do not know the effects of vaccinating with the new ones; but according to their package inserts, about 2% of students receiving them will be sickened or hospitalized with a serious adverse event—i.e., an additional 8,000 sick students and 24 deaths—for a total of 12,000 sick and 36 dead, in the attempt to possibly avert three meningitis cases and one death.[7]

In addition, none of this takes into account its still largely undocumented share of brain damage and chronic autoimmune diseases, which are often slower to develop and to that extent mostly written off, as we saw. But even the official statistics are already quite sufficient to invalidate the rationale for its use, let alone for requiring it.

HEPATITIS A

In the United States, hepatitis A is also uncommon, currently averaging about 3,000 cases annually, according to the CDC.[8] It is almost entirely an acute infection, which is rarely fatal, and complete recovery is the rule, although in very rare instances it can result in acute liver failure and death. In children under 6, it is often asymptomatic, and only about 10% develop jaundice; but in older children and adolescents the disease is usually more severe, and over 70% of the cases become jaundiced.[9] Currently, the vaccine is mandated for small children in day care, elementary, and secondary school in 20 states.[10]

The CDC estimates the death rate from hepatitis A at 3–6 per 1,000 cases,[11] which adds up to approximately 9–18 deaths per year. Once again, the rationale for vaccinating everybody against a disease that very few people will get and fewer than 20 will die from rests upon the widespread assumption that vaccines are essentially harmless, so that it is perfectly safe to pile on as many as we wish, which is ironically contradicted by the Supreme Court's ruling that they are "unavoidably unsafe," not to mention the variety and extent of serious adverse reactions that we have already discussed.

Thus even the *PDR* lists several of the usual autoimmune type that we've come to expect: convulsions, anaphylaxis, encephalopathy, Guillain-Barré syndrome, multiple sclerosis, neuropathy, myelitis, dyspnea, erythema multiforme, angioedema, thrombocytopenia, and menstrual disorders.[12] In addition, both the GlaxoSmithKline and Merck vaccines (Havrix and Vaqta, respectively) list the following ingredients with either well-established or highly probable toxicity:

aluminum hydroxide, amorphous aluminum hydroxyphosphate sulfate, formaldehyde, MRC-5 lung fibroblasts from an aborted male fetus, bovine albumin, and neomycin.[13] So once again, Professor Gordon Stewart's criterion appears to have been satisfied, that the risk of serious adverse effects far exceeds the risk of anything comparable from the disease, or indeed of catching it to begin with.

HUMAN PAPILLOMA VIRUS (HPV)

Like the hepatitis B vaccines, those directed against the human papilloma virus, or HPV, are recombinant or bioengineered versions of the virus, with all the attendant problems thereof; it is also the first vaccine whose ultimate target is not the virus itself, as much as the noninfectious disease sometimes associated with it, namely, cancer of the cervix.

According to the National Cancer Institute, an NIH affiliate, approximately 13,000 women will develop cervical cancer in 2016, and some 4,100 are likely to die of it;[14] but 14 million Americans are newly infected with the virus every year; and roughly 50% of all sexually active men and 80% of all sexually active women will become infected with at least one serotype in their lifetime,[15] while the incidence of cervical cancer, thanks in large part to preventive screening, has continued to decline precipitously.

The original HPV vaccine was directed against serotypes 16 and 18, which are associated with approximately 70% of all cervical cancer cases; and the latest version has added seven more serotypes thought to confer somewhat higher risk;[16] but a 2014 study showed that naturally acquired antibodies to types 16 and 18 are in fact *protective* against cervical cancer,[17] a finding that argues against trying to imitate the natural process by artificial and potentially hazardous means, not to mention the fact that cervical screening tests, such as the Pap smear, have already lowered the incidence and mortality rates of cervical cancer by at least 80%.[18]

Furthermore, as we know, it is only a matter of time before these HPV vaccines, to the extent they are effective, will simply have shifted the risk of cervical cancer to other serotypes, as is already occurring with so many other vaccines. The same is also likely to be true for anal, oropharyngeal, and penile cancer, which are similarly linked to sexually transmitted HPV infection, especially by type 16.[19]

But the strongest case to be made against the HPV vaccines is their appalling record of death and serious injuries, which surpasses even the influenza and hepatitis B, such that even the pious assurances of the CDC and the vaccine establishment have not been entirely successful in keeping it from the headlines. To begin with, these vaccines are bioengineered, and therefore need aluminum-salt adjuvants to achieve significant antigenicity; in addition, they contain other potentially dangerous and as yet untested ingredients that we have already discussed, such as insect cell and viral proteins, bacterial cell proteins, yeast proteins, and the detergent polysorbate 80.[20]

Second, even by the CDC's improbably low estimate of 3–4 serious adverse events per 100,000 doses, the risk of the vaccine is at least comparable to the death rate from cervical cancer;[21] and we know that the actual risk from the vaccine is much higher than that, not only because adverse events are massively underreported, as we saw, but also because the retrospective CDC study uncritically accepted the manufacturer's minimalist safety criteria.[22] The neuroscientists Tomljenovic and Shaw sum up the equation admirably:

> All drugs are associated with some risks of adverse reactions. Because vaccines are given to the healthy, the uncertainty of benefit means that only a small level of risk is acceptable. Furthermore, medical ethics demand that vaccination be carried out with the participants' full, informed consent, based on objective disclosure of known and foreseeable benefits and risks.
>
> While leading medical authorities state that HPV vaccines are important for preventing cervical cancer, clinical trials show no evidence supporting that conclusion. Similarly, contrary to claims that cervical cancer is common worldwide, in the West it is increasingly rare, with mortality rates several times lower than the rate of deaths and serious adverse reactions from the vaccine.[23]

As a footnote to the above, fully informed consent is obviously impossible when vaccines are required by law of everyone, unless potential recipients retain the right of refusal, as in a personal-belief exemption or something like it.

Finally, one of the most distinctive features of both HPV vaccines is that an unprecedented number of deaths and serious adverse reactions in teenage girls have been reported in the news since they were first introduced, breaking through the largely self-imposed media blackout for a change.

In the UK, where the vaccine has been given routinely to an estimated 8 million 12- and 13-year-old girls since 2008, an article in the London *Daily Express* noted that over 8,200 had reported "debilitating side effects," notably chest and abdominal pain, exhaustion, fainting, shortness of breath, tachycardia, and fibromyalgia, more than one-fourth of which were considered "life-threatening" and required emergency treatment in the ER, and that these figures were generally agreed to represent no more than 10% of the actual number.[24]

In the Gardasil package insert, the following adverse reactions are listed as having been reported to the VAERS system, including many of the usual suspects, but also quite a few more:

1. cellulitis;
2. autoimmune hemolytic anemia, idiopathic thrombocytopenic purpura, lymphadenopathy;
3. nausea, vomiting, pancreatitis;
4. asthenia, chills, fatigue, malaise;
5. autoimmune hypersensitivity reactions, anaphylaxis, bronchospasm, and urticaria;
6. arthralgias and myalgias:
7. acute disseminated encephalomyelitis, vertigo, Guillain-Barré syndrome, headache, motor neuron disease, paralysis, seizures, syncope (with tonic-clonic movements, other seizure-like activity, and falls and injuries), and transverse myelitis.;
8. deep venous thrombosis, pulmonary embolus; and
9. death.[25]

Of particular interest was the unexpected frequency of syncope, or fainting, which later studies identified as postural orthostatic tachycardia syndrome, or POTS, a condition of tachycardia and fainting on standing up, indicating an autonomic nervous system dysfunction.[26] Even more disturbing was the recent finding of prolonged amenorrhea and premature menopause due to ovarian failure in young adolescent girls, putting an end to their hopes of giving birth,[27] which has alarmed gynecologists and pediatricians alike, and prompted an official warning from the American College of Pediatricians of a possible link to ovarian cancer.[28]

Other reports of ALS,[29] or Lou Gehrig's disease, and an unprecedented number of deaths in girls and boys seemingly in the prime of health,[30] have continued to shock the nation. In one such case, DNA fragments from HPV type 16 were demonstrated in the dead girl's blood and spleen at autopsy, a finding which not only dispelled any lingering doubts as to causation, but was also potentially relevant to other cases written off as "coincidental," because she died suddenly in her sleep fully six months after her last injection.[31]

In any case, probably due in no small part to its application to a largely benign infection, a target population of adolescent girls at the beginning of their reproductive life, and a disease largely on the decline in the developed world, the HPV vaccines have not as yet been welcomed with much enthusiasm by either the medical community or the general public, with at least 27% of pediatricians and family doctors declining to recommend them strongly, routinely, or at all,[32] despite intense lobbying by the ACIP, the CDC, and the industry. So far, only Rhode Island, Virginia, and the District of Columbia have agreed to mandate it.

Finally, the manufacturers' aggressive marketing tactics, including paying large sums to researchers to promote the vaccines and the systematic cover-up of side effects, have driven a number of senior scientists involved in their development to publicly repudiate the industry's policies and at least implicitly regret their own participation in them.

The first of these was Dr. Diane Harper, who helped design the Phase II and III safety and efficacy trials for both Gardasil and Cervarix, and expressed many of the same reservations articulated by Tomljenovic and Shaw, namely, that the trials were invalid, that cervical cancer has been effectively controlled with preventive screening and early detection, and that the risk of adverse reactions already exceeded the risk of the disease.[33] In a 2014 interview with the French magazine *Principes de Santé,* Dr. Bernard Dalbergue, yet another former Merck employee, went even further:

> Everyone knew when this vaccine was released on the American market that it would prove worthless! Gardasil costs a fortune, is useless, and decision-makers at all levels are aware of it! I predict that it will become the greatest medical scandal of all time, because the evidence will add up that this vaccine, technical and scientific feat though it may be, has absolutely no effect on cervical cancer, and that all the very many adverse effects which destroy lives and even kill serve no other purpose than to generate profit for the manufacturers. There is far too much financial interest for these medicines to be withdrawn.[34]

In many countries of Europe and from around the world, these vaccines have occasioned numerous investigations, lawsuits, and government bans, as the result of a shocking number of deaths and permanent disabilities, and an unprecedented volume of negative publicity.

In 2013, the Japanese government officially withdrew its recommendation of Gardasil, based on 2,000 adverse reactions reported in just 3 years, including seizures, brain damage, blindness, paralysis, memory loss, speech impairment, and pancreatitis, not to mention its exorbitant cost of $600 per dose.[35] According to the *Tokyo Times*, Japanese health authorities placed the blame squarely on the American government for covering up the risks and persuading other countries to accept it on that basis: "Not only does the Obama administration continue recommending the vaccine; it spends large sums of taxpayer dollars in promoting it, and works hard to keep its dangers secret."[36]

Meanwhile, attorneys in Japan, India, Spain, Denmark, France, and other nations have done what the US Supreme Court has enjoined their American counterparts from doing, namely, filing lawsuits for damages against HPV vaccine manufacturers on behalf of their victims.

In Spain, the suit names Merck and Sanofi-Pasteur for manipulating and falsifying data, as well as federal and provincial health authorities for ignoring widespread calls for a moratorium on the vaccines until these issues are resolved; the full list of charges, encompassing the very issues we have been discussing, reads as follows:

1. fraudulent marketing and/or administration of an inadequately tested vaccine;
2. failure to inform the public about the potential risks of Gardasil;
3. infringement of the right to informed consent;
4. ignoring new medical conditions in the recipients in spite of their similarity and the short period of time between the vaccination and the onset of symptoms;
5. ignoring scientific evidence of the harmful effects of Gardasil ingredients and methods of manufacture;
6. callous disregard for those suffering from reactions to Gardasil;
7. failure to inform the public that HPV infections are only one risk factor for cervical cancer;
8. failure to inform the public that 90% of all HPV infections clear on their own without medical intervention;
9. failure to inform the public about alternative methods of controlling cervical cancer; and
10. criminal liability for injuries resulting from vaccination with Gardasil.[37]

In Denmark, a documentary that aired on national television quoted a number of prominent Danish physicians who testified that, based on their experience, adverse reactions to Gardasil were several orders of magnitude higher than they had been led to expect.[38]

One such was Dr. Jasper Mehlsen, a specialist at the Fredriksberg Hospital, who had personally vaccinated over 3,000 adolescent girls, cared for many of those with serious complications, and reported a waiting list of 6–9 months before new victims could be properly evaluated: "We thought the rate of serious adverse events was about 1 in 10,000; now a realistic estimate is that 1 in 500 girls, or 1,000 of the 500,000 who were vaccinated, will experience serious side effects."[39]

A colleague, Dr. Stig Gerdes, feared that the numbers will climb still higher: "It will not surprise me if we end up reaching several thousand who are sick. I stopped using Gardasil a few years ago, after vaccinating just 100 patients. More than a handful of them became ill, several of them very, very seriously."[40]

In India, a group of aggrieved parents charged that several of their children died from receiving Gardasil and Cervarix without their consent, as part of a 2015 trial funded by the Bill and Melinda Gates Foundation, after a Parliamentary investigation found that the trials involved "a clear violation of medical ethics and basic human rights, amounting to child abuse"; and the Indian Supreme Court ordered the Indian government to explain the conduct of these trials, their monitoring of adverse effects, and their policy on liability and compensation for the victims.[41]

In Colombia, when hundreds of adolescent girls suddenly developed mysterious illnesses after being given recently mandated HPV vaccines, their mothers and friends took to the streets in several major cities, demanding that the government

- provide medical care for the roughly 800 girls affected so far;
- conduct studies to determine the exact causes of these illnesses; and
- suspend further use of HPV vaccines until these things were done.[42]

At the Third Colombian Symposium on Autoimmunity, which happened to coincide with these demonstrations, Professor Yehuda Shoenfeld rejected the possibility that this strange flurry of illnesses could be a kind of "mass hysteria," as some pro-vaccine advocates had suggested:

> It is very unlikely that the symptoms presented after receiving the vaccine are due to psychological reasons. Elsewhere in the world, the vaccine produces the same signs and symptoms as in the girls; and when we gave it to mice, they did also. We have to ask whether the vaccine is really needed; if the negative effects outweigh the benefits, it should not be given.

> We believe that aluminum is toxic for the brain. Experimental research shows clearly that aluminum adjuvants have a potential for inducing serious immunological disorders in humans, and for autoimmunity in particular, with inflammation of the brain, long-term neurological complications, and thus profound consequences for health.[43]

Once again, the most thoughtful and clearheaded review of all the evidence regarding HPV vaccines came from the neuroscientists Tomljenovic and Shaw,[44] who pointed out the following:

1. Merck, the CDC, the American Academy of Pediatrics, and the AMA aggressively promoted Gardasil as safe and effective long before the appropriate studies were completed.[45]
2. It received FDA Fast-Track approval to fulfill an unmet need when the Pap test screening had already reduced cervical cancer deaths by 70%.[46]
3. Its touted five-year effectiveness in reducing cervical intraepithelial neoplasia (CIN) is undercut by the fact that almost all CIN's reverse themselves spontaneously in any case.[47]
4. Thirty-five percent of girls and women vaccinated showed no detectable antibodies after five years.[48]
5. Between 2006 and 2012, the VAERS system received 21,265 reports of adverse reactions to Gardasil, of which 9,565 involved ER visits, 1,669 were serious, 609 permanently disabling, 363 life threatening, 212 needed long-term hospitalization, and 78 were fatal.[49]
6. Of all vaccinations in women under 30, Gardasil alone accounted for more than 60% of all serious adverse reactions, 61.9% of all deaths, 64.9% of all life-threatening reactions, and 81.8% of all permanent disabilities.[50]
7. Its safety trials involved the use of aluminum-containing "placebo" even though aluminum salts are a known neurotoxin and have been implicated in ASIA and various forms of brain damage.[51]
8. It has not yet been proven effective in preventing cervical cancer.[52]

VACCINES IN THE PIPELINE

In a 2013 press release from the drug industry's promotional website, more than 270 new vaccines were said to be already in development, either at various stages of the clinical trial process or under FDA review, including "137 for infectious diseases, 99 for cancer, 15 for allergies, and 10 for neurological disorders,"[53] such as a vaccine against HIV, "to delay disease progression"; monoclonal-antibody vaccines "against pandemic and seasonal influenza"; a "genetically modified vaccine designed for treatment" of pancreatic cancer; and an "irradiated vaccine" for protection against malaria.[54]

DNA VACCINES AND GENE TRANSFER

Vaccines against many of the emerging infectious diseases, like Ebola, dengue, chikungunya, Zika, SARS, and West Nile virus are already in the works; as acute infections primarily, these represent new applications of the same technology that we have had for a long time, for stimulating the humoral mechanism to produce antibodies against the invading foreign organism.

For chronic infections, however, like Lyme disease, malaria, TB, hepatitis C, and HIV, vaccines designed in the old way to produce antibodies against the organism have so far proved ineffective. Working more or less independently of one another, a number of scientists have been experimenting with a radically new technology called immunoprophylaxis by gene transfer, or IGT, which delivers synthetic new genes into the DNA of the recipient that have been bioengineered to be resistant to HIV, for example, and will thus supposedly help AIDS patients to eliminate the virus and protect themselves from reinfection in the future.[55] According to the esteemed science writer Carl Zimmer,

> This treatment is not a vaccine in an ordinary sense. By delivering synthetic genes into the muscles of the monkeys, the scientists are essentially re-engineering the animals themselves to resist disease. Researchers are testing this novel approach not just against HIV, but also Ebola, malaria, influenza and hepatitis. "The sky's the limit," said Michael Farzan, an immunologist at Scripps, who hopes that this technique may provide long-term protection against diseases for which vaccines have failed.[56]

In their 2008 article for *Medscape*, "The Emerging Role of DNA Vaccines," Drs. McDonnell and Askari of the University of Michigan were among the first to describe the process:

> Vaccines composed of DNA are injected into subjects whose own cellular machinery translates the nucleotide sequences into peptides [simple amino-

acid or protein-like chains of low molecular weight], which are capable of inducing a brisk *cellular* immune response, in contrast with traditional vaccines, which induce mainly a *humoral* response.

As yet there are no such vaccines on the market, and no published data showing efficacy in humans. While these studies have only just begun, the concepts behind them have dramatically changed the way many in the basic sciences are approaching their work. A vaccine that stimulates an effective cellular immune response could be used to treat patients already infected with chronic viral illnesses, such as HIV or hepatitis C, and also to fight cancer cells.

DNA vaccines differ from recombinant vaccines [like Hepatitis B or HPV] in that the immunogenic protein in the latter is made in the laboratory, whereas in the DNA vaccine it is synthesized within the cells of the host.[57]

On the face of it, the idea of stimulating the cellular immune system sounds appealing, because the limited focus of traditional vaccines on antibody production was thought by many critics to weaken the more fundamental cellular mechanisms, as we saw. On the other hand, as Dr. Zimmer pointed out, DNA vaccines are not really vaccines at all, but rather foreign DNA that has been genetically engineered to provoke a cellular immune response in the host in the form of a highly antigenic foreign protein, which could easily trigger an even wider variety of autoimmune responses if the new DNA were actually incorporated into the genetic material of the host. According to McDonnell and Askari,

> There are many potential problems and unanswered questions. The possibility of mutagenesis needs to be rigorously tested. There is no evidence that the new DNA integrates into the host genome; but if it did, it would raise the specter of carcinogenesis, of turning on cancer genes or turning off tumor-suppressing ones. What if the new DNA circulated throughout the body and became integrated into germ cells? Might not later generations express the antigen from birth and thus develop tolerance rather than immunity to it? Anti-DNA antibody formation and autoimmune diseases are other possibilities.[58]

Six years later, when Dr. Zimmer wrote his piece on the new technology, these questions were still unanswered: "Whether IGT will succeed is still an open question. Researchers still need to gauge its safety and effectiveness in humans. And the prospect of genetically engineering people to resist infectious diseases may raise concerns among patients."[59]

That's putting it mildly. For me, and for other practicing physicians whose knowledge of and curiosity about science and the natural world are shaped and tempered by knowing and treating real people, this Brave New World sounds even scarier than the one we already inhabit. Here are the thoughts of Catherine Shanahan, MD, a board-certified family doctor with over twenty years of clinical experience, and additional training in biochemistry and genetics, who tackles the issue in her blog:

> Recently I heard about a new biotechnology for making DNA Vaccines. The thought of it makes my blood run cold. What they're talking about is turning people into genetically modified organisms. Regular vaccines inoculate recipients with the same proteins they would be exposed to anyway, if infected with the virus in question. DNA vaccines work by altering our own DNA, by changing us at a cellular level.
>
> DNA vaccines deliver the DNA into the nucleus of the muscle cell itself, forcing it to produce viral proteins, potentially for the rest of your life. According to the Indian biochemist Neeraj Kumar, "extended immunostimulation leads to chronic inflammation," potentially to a serious auto-immune disorder like lupus or myasthenia gravis.[60]

SUMMARY

The present generation of vaccines features three that have already been mandated, or are in the process of being mandated, in many states, namely, those against meningococcal disease, hepatitis A, and HPV.

Like the Hib and pneumococcus, the meningococcus vaccines are *conjugates*, incorporating tetanus or diphtheria toxoid for greater antigencity, and involving other ingredients known to be toxic, like formaldehyde, as well as others that have not yet been investigated, but should be, like proteins derived from beef, yeast, and bioengineered *E. coli.* Although meningococcal disease is often serious and sometimes fatal, it is distinctly rare, while the vaccine has been linked to the usual quota of autoimmune diseases, so that vaccinating everyone against it seems not only unnecessary, but ill-advised, offering casualties far in excess of any possible benefit.

With the hepatitis A vaccine, the cost-benefit analysis is even more unfavorable. In addition to being similarly uncommon, the disease is very rarely fatal or even serious, especially in children, and almost everyone recovers from it completely, without complications or sequelae, while the vaccine is ineffective without aluminum adjuvants, with their well-known propensity to cause brain damage and other autoimmune diseases. I see no compelling reason for using it at all, let alone requiring it of all children.

But for minimal benefit and maximum risk, the HPV vaccines, Gardasil and Cervarix, are in a class by themselves. Like the Hep B, they are recombinant (i.e., genetically engineered), require aluminum adjuvants, and also contain many other ingredients deserving further scrutiny, namely, insect cell and viral proteins, bacterial cell proteins, yeast proteins, and the detergent polysorbate 80. Furthermore, its intended target is not the HPV virus itself, which is ubiquitous, almost always benign and self-limiting, and antibodies against which are actually protective, but rather cervical cancer, its increasingly uncommon complication, of which preventive screening alone has already reduced the incidence and mortality by 80%.

In addition, it is intended mainly for prepubescent children and adolescents of both sexes, before they begin their sexual and reproductive lives, against a disease that takes 20–40 years to develop; and it has caused not only premature menopause and ovarian failure, but also so many deaths and disabling complications that a number of countries in Europe, Asia, and Latin America are no longer recommending its use, and have filed suits against the manufacturers on behalf of victims.

Beyond these three, at least dozens and probably hundreds of new vaccines are already in development, no doubt encouraged by the old belief that they are completely safe, so that it is perfectly all right to add on as many as we like, and by the continuing absence of any serious regulation or restraint.

In addition to vaccines against acute diseases of global import, such as SARS, Ebola, dengue, chikungunya, and Zika, new DNA technology has opened a path for experimentation against chronic diseases, such as Lyme disease, TB, malaria, herpes, hepatitis C, and various forms of cancer, for which traditional vaccines have so far proved ineffective. Unlike the vaccines we are familiar with, the new technology is really a form of gene transfer, in which DNA that has been modified to attack a certain virus or bacterium is introduced directly into the host, whose native DNA then translates that foreign characteristic into a highly antigenic peptide, such that the resulting immune response involves both cellular and humoral components. On the other hand, the risk of permanently altering the host's DNA in the process seems almost certain to frighten the general public even more than they already are, especially since the science remains as yet poorly understood, and the investigation of these risks is still in an early stage.

PART V

CONCLUSION

Chapter 14

WHERE TO GO FROM HERE

OK, that's the evidence. In this concluding chapter, I want to think about what ties it all together, what follows from it, and what actions are indicated and most appropriate to undertake at this point.

A SACRAMENT OF MODERN MEDICINE

Ever since I became interested in and concerned about vaccines, I've been struck by their uniquely privileged status in our society, which cannot be written off entirely to the greed of the manufacturers and the lust for power of the government agencies and physicians who advocate for them, even though if not precisely because these twin motives have proved so pervasive and so improbably successful in this instance.

By the standards of contemporary science, the principles of justice and morality, and the dictates of logic and common sense alike, our present policies regarding vaccination are incoherent and indeed self-contradictory in several mutually reinforcing respects. In the first place, the industry is allowed to dispense with well-established scientific standards like the use of placebo-controlled trials, and even to violate basic ethical norms, such as providing fully informed consent, proclaimed as a universal human right in both the Nuremberg Code and the Helsinki Declaration,[1] even while continuing to affirm its solemn commitment to these same principles.

In addition, the CDC regularly assures the public that vaccines are uniformly safe, having arbitrarily ruled out any adverse effects occurring after a few days; yet the Supreme Court has ruled that they are inherently *unsafe*, in order to shield the manufacturers from liability for the injuries they cause, so that their victims are required by law to receive them, but no longer have the right to sue them for damages in court, to which every other industry is subject.

Vaccines are widely regarded as safe and effective by virtual consensus of the American medical and scientific communities, and are accepted without question or demur by large segments of the general public, while ignoring a large and growing body of scientific evidence to the contrary; yet children are required by law to receive them, with or without their parents' consent, and often without detailed and accurate information about their risks, with the result that both children and adults are routinely subjected to a heavier vaccine burden than those of any other country on earth, with no compelling public health emergency anywhere in sight.

These are a few of the more glaring inconsistencies, which we have already explored in detail; I list them again merely to show that no combination of the basic principles of science, economics, morality, and simple common sense can suffice to make a coherent case for our present policy of requiring everyone to be vaccinated, even against their will if necessary.

To them, I would add two more that are equally striking but less often appreciated, namely, the dutiful self-censorship of the news media, which seemingly never have to be told to refrain from saying anything derogatory about vaccines, and the readiness of most physicians to offer up their own children for the same vaccines that they administer to their patients.

Finally, to me perhaps the most telling example of all is the crusading zeal underlying the successful public-relations campaigns that eventually persuaded the vast majority of practicing doctors and their patients to go along with the chicken pox, rotavirus, and flu vaccines, even though by the vaccine establishment's own admission they are directed against illnesses that almost everyone recovers from, will save only a few dozen or at most a hundred lives per year, and by their own impossibly understated figures have already caused at least that many deaths and permanently disabling injuries.

Taken together, all of these supremely uneconomical enthusiasms bear witness to a sincere, reverent, virtually universal, and essentially blind faith in the safety and efficacy of vaccines, as a kind of baptismal initiation into what Bob Mendelsohn and others have aptly called the religion of modern medicine.[2] As sacraments of our faith, they need no longer conform to the rules and requirements of science, logic, economics, ethics, and common sense that most other countries insist upon, even while their most zealous proponents continue to pledge undying allegiance to them. This is *scientism*, a quasi-religious dogmatism in the name of science, the main result of which is to stifle the critical thinking, questioning, and doubting of settled truths that true science requires, as perfectly captured by René Dubos, the great microbiologist:

> Faith in the magical power of drugs often blunts the critical senses, and comes close at times to a mass hysteria, involving scientists and laymen alike. Men want miracles as much today as in the past. If they do not join one of the newer cults, they satisfy this need by worshiping at the altar of modern science. This faith is not new. It has helped to give medicine the authority of a priesthood, and to recreate the glamor of ancient mysteries.[3]

TRUTH AND SELF-CENSORSHIP IN THE MEDIA

Ever since becoming involved with this issue almost forty years ago, I have never ceased to wonder at the virtually complete absence of news stories—whether in print or on the radio or TV—that report a case of vaccine injury as an actual occurrence in the same objective, value-neutral tone as a fire, theft, or murder in the neighborhood, attesting as well as anything else to the uncommonly high degree of awe and esteem accorded to vaccines in American society. In 1993, at the beginning of the Clinton era, I noticed a front-page item in the *Boston Globe* that let the cat out of the bag just this once:

> **INOCULATIONS PUT ASPIN IN THE HOSPITAL.**
> Defense Secretary Les Aspin was in "improved" condition but remained in the ICU of Georgetown University Hospital after suffering breathing difficulties after routine inoculations. While "definitely on the road to recovery," he remained in the ICU to be monitored, because he has a history of heart problems, and fluid collected in his lungs. He entered the hospital because of shortness of breath aggravated by "a mild, pre-existing heart condition," the Pentagon said. He became ill the day before, soon after receiving a number of immunization shots for travel abroad.[4]

Although Aspin's hospitalization for congestive heart failure remained newsworthy for several more days, there was no further mention of his vaccinations, so that readers who missed the original story were given the impression that he merely suffered a flare-up of his preexisting heart condition, as was indeed the case, thus admirably illustrating both the nonspecific effect of the vaccination process that I have been at such pains to describe, and the synergistic effect of receiving several vaccinations at once.

Seemingly without having to be told, the news media likewise habitually protect themselves by simply quoting the parents, which allows them to sympathize with their grief, and even their belief that their child's death or disabling injury was caused by vaccines, without ever accepting that linkage as settled fact.

Similarly, in medical journals reporting on outbreaks of measles, mumps, pertussis, and the like, it has been and still remains a common practice to omit the important statistic of how many cases had previously been vaccinated, since a high percentage would imply that the vaccine was ineffective, and thus possibly jeopardize the CDC's cherished goal of maximum compliance.

In many such outbreaks, as we saw, it turns out that a large majority of the cases, quite often even 95% or more, had in fact been vaccinated according to the approved CDC schedule, as had the local population as a whole. In other examples, where the percentage of vaccinated cases was reported to be somewhat lower, there would often be a sizable fraction, perhaps 20–30%, whose vaccination status was listed as "unknown," a reference to parents who claimed that their children had been vaccinated but hadn't been told or thought it necessary to bring their documents to prove it.

With the addition of more and more new vaccines since the 1990s, however, these unspoken taboos and the quasi-religious veneration that impelled the media to observe them have slowly begun to weaken. A few courageous investigative reporters, like Sharyl Attkisson at *CBS News* (and later independently), have doggedly pursued the vaccine-autism linkage, for example, and the scandalous role of the industry and the CDC in covering it up, as in this commentary she posted on her blog:

> A new study this week found no link between vaccines and autism. It instantly made headlines on TV news and popular media everywhere. Many billed it as the final word, once again disproving the notion that vaccines had anything to do with autism. What you didn't learn on the news was that the study was from a consulting firm that lists major vaccine makers among its clients. That potential conflict of interest was not disclosed in the paper published in *The New England Journal of Medicine.*
>
> When the popular press, bloggers and medical pundits uncritically promote a study like this one, it must confound researchers whose peer-reviewed, published works have found possible links between vaccines and autism. But their research has not been endorsed and promoted by the government, and therefore

has not been widely reported in the media. In fact, news reports, blogs, and "medical experts" routinely claim that no such studies exist.[5]

In recent years, the Internet, social media, and blogosphere have similarly provided ready platforms for thousands upon thousands of parents of vaccine-injured children, their friends and supporters, and for doctors, nurses, scientists, and other health professionals, all struggling to be heard above the clamor of official propaganda and the even more deafening silence of the self-imposed media blackout. Collectively they attest to a vast infrastructure of protest and dissent that shares personal stories, mounts demonstrations at state legislatures and CDC headquarters, and does the necessary homework for uncovering neglected research.

One such site is Stop Mandatory Vaccination, stopmandatoryvaccination.com, which advocates for free choice about vaccines, and solicits and publicizes personal stories of the vaccine-injured, among other public-spirited activities.[6]

In 2015, when the California legislature approved SB277 eliminating the personal-belief exemption, and the bill sat on Governor Brown's desk awaiting his imprimatur, this group along with many others mounted demonstrations opposing it all across the state; day after day, week after week, thousands kept showing up at the State House in Sacramento to protest it, as well as calling press conferences and inviting sympathetic doctors and legislators to speak out on their behalf.[7] When Governor Brown eventually signed it into law, another group instantly materialized out of nowhere and filed a lawsuit seeking to overturn it, organized by the mother of yet another vaccine-injured child.[8]

In countless similar incidents involving groups and events both local and national, the movement for safer vaccines, informed consent, and parental choice continues to grow, still largely under the radar of the mainstream media, but already in sufficient numbers to begin to dispel the aura of sanctity surrounding both the theory and practice of vaccination.

Analogous developments are also under way within the medical and nursing professions themselves, indicating a growing skepticism that has at least tempered, moderated, and smoothed off the rough edges of the official stance of vaccinating everybody against everything at every possible opportunity. Thus, as we saw, sizable numbers of practicing physicians are refusing to give their own children certain vaccinations, or to vaccinate them at the officially recommended time.

Unsurprisingly, such noncompliance is far more prevalent in Europe, where vaccines are generally regarded more soberly as simply another medical procedure, without the religious overtones. One study of Swiss pediatricians, for example, discovered that 32% shied away from the Hep B vaccines, and 29% from the Hib, while only 13% gave their own kids flu shots, only 5% the pneumococcus, and only 3% the chicken pox.[9]

Even in the United States, where the religious dimension is more prominent than anywhere else, a 2008 CDC-funded study found that 11% of pediatricians and family physicians no longer urge parents to give their children all the recommended vaccines, and that family doctors were substantially more likely than pediatricians to deviate from the official policy and to voice concerns about vaccine safety.[10]

In some areas, while it is still fairly common for pediatricians and FPs to refuse to care for children whose parents want to pick and choose, a growing number are allowing such parents to customize their children's vaccine schedule, and even to decide *not* to give some or all of them, without terminating the relationship or disrespecting their right to choose, even when they strongly disagree and perhaps even argue with them about it. While support for vaccination remains strong among most physicians, the willingness of the younger generation especially to let parents have the say indicates a growing awareness that too many vaccines are being promoted for less than compelling reasons, and suggests that a kinder, gentler future may not be too far off.

Even higher rates of noncompliance have been observed among nurses, whose duties include actually administering the shots, and many of whom are also being forced to accept the flu and sometimes the Hep B vaccine themselves as conditions of their employment. In a 2009 survey involving 1,017 American RNs, for example, 41% of the respondents had declined their flu shot during the previous season, citing concerns about adverse reactions and lack of effectiveness.[11] In 2014, a group of 22,000 nurses was formed in states and localities all over the country, calling itself Nurses against Mandatory Vaccines, or NAMV, to protest against hospitals requiring flu shots for their employees:

> Experienced nurses across the US are choosing to lose their jobs rather than submit to mandatory flu vaccinations. Dreonna Breton, a Pennsylvania R.N., recently refused the vaccine because she was pregnant, with a history of miscarriages, and her doctor advised her against it; but her hospital fired her anyway. Nurses granted exemptions are forced to wear masks for the entire flu season, even though studies have shown that those vaccinated still pass on the virus.[12]

Later that same year, the Massachusetts Nurses Association filed suit against Brigham and Women's Hospital in Boston for instituting the same requirement, and Trish Powers, one of the Brigham nurses, issued a public statement explaining their reasons:

> I am proud to be a nurse at Brigham and Women's Hospital. But the flu vaccine is only 59% effective, and carries with it serious health risks, which are not disclosed to those receiving it. As of November 2013, the VAERS Reporting System has received 93,000 reports of adverse reactions, hospitalizations, injuries and deaths following influenza vaccinations, including 1,080 deaths, 8,888 hospitalizations and 1,811 disabilities. Nurses are more aware of this data than the general public, and many of us don't feel that the low effectiveness rate of the vaccine warrants the health risk.[13]

Because they are much more intimately involved in the physical details of patient care, nurses have also been especially prominent and outspoken in the movement for safer vaccines in general, and in support of parents' right to choose.

Modest though they are, I cite these developments to show that slowly and incrementally, the privileged and indeed worshipful status widely accorded to vaccines is being challenged by increasing numbers of parents, doctors, and nurses on behalf of the general public, a trend giving grounds for hope that these drugs will one day be made to run the gauntlet of objective scientific scrutiny, like any other medical procedure, rather than excused from criticism by the trappings of religion and rubber-stamped by the agencies meant to regulate them.

THE MORE, THE MERRIER

In the catechism of vaccination, a central article of faith is that the vaccines are essentially safe and uniformly effective, as we saw, so that

1. the few, rare adverse reactions that are legitimate must satisfy the strictest possible standards for causation and be limited to this or that individual vaccine;
2. it is unnecessary, if not blasphemous, to study the possible ill effects of the vaccination process *per se;* and
3. echoing the theology of Dr. Offit, it is entirely permissible and even desirable to pile on as many doses of as many different vaccines as we like.

The scientific and clinical evidence already presented is more than sufficient to establish precisely the opposite conclusion, 1) that vaccinations are inherently and significantly linked to illness and death, are indeed "unavoidably unsafe," in Justice Scalia's felicitous phrase, and 2) that these risks are tied less directly to *which* particular vaccines are given, than simply to *how many*, that is, to the total vaccine *load.*

For children and adolescents, from birth to 18 years of age, the ACIP's recommended schedule for 2016 reads as follows:

2016 Recommended Immunization Schedule (0–18 Years of Age)[14]		
Hepatitis B	3 doses: at birth, 1–2 months, and 6–18 months	3
Rotavirus	3 doses: 2, 4, and 6 months (RotaTeq)	3
DTaP	5 doses: 2, 4, 6 months; 15–18 months; 4–6 years	5
Hib	4 doses: 2, 4, 6 months; 12–15 months	4
Pneumococcus	4 doses: 2, 4, 6 months; 12–15 months	4
Polio (IPV)	4 doses: 2, 4 months; 6–18 months; 4–6 years	4
Influenza	16–22 doses: 1–2 yearly till age 6; 1 yearly thereafter	19
MMR	2 doses: 12–15 months; 4–6 years	2
Chicken pox	2 doses: 12–15 months; 4–6 years	2
Hepatitis A	2 doses: 12–24 months	2
Meningococcus	2 doses: 11–12 years; 16–18 years	2
Tdap	1 dose: 11–12 years	1
HPV	3 doses: 11–12 years	3

This adds up to 54 vaccine doses by the time a child enters college; and since the MMR, DTaP, and Tdap each contain three separate components, that adds 16 more doses for a total load of 70 doses of individual vaccine components. In addition, many of these vaccines are given simultaneously at the same visit, like the DTaP, Hib, pneumo, and IPV (six components), or the MMR and chicken pox (four components), and so forth, a time-saving convenience that itself, we now know, confers a significantly increased risk of death and serious, life-threatening injuries.

And this is just the beginning. After decades of open season on our children, in recent years, the industry, their physician-advocates, and the CDC have increasingly sought to extend their dominion over the entire population, including mature adults, the middle-aged, the elderly, and even pregnant women, as we have seen, chiefly by aggressive marketing to physicians. The campaign to vaccinate adults began in earnest during the Clinton years, when traditional warnings and contraindications were increasingly superseded and swept aside by cost-benefit calculations, as we saw.

In the 1996 article "Adult Immunizations: How Are We Doing?," a typical example of the genre, a leading infectious disease specialist calculated the number of lives that could be saved by vaccinating adults with the same zeal and thoroughness that we had previously reserved for our children:

> 30,000 lives could be saved every year if adult immunization recommendations were implemented. Between 50,000 and 70,000 people die annually from influenza, pneumococcal infection, and hepatitis B. This exceeds the number of automobile deaths, and far outweighs mortality from these same diseases in children. Those for whom vaccines are contraindicated are fewer than those who fail to be immunized on account of the following, which are not contraindications but often thought to be:
>
> 1. local reactions to previous vaccines, including fever less than 104°;
> 2. a mild acute illness, with or without fever;
> 3. antibiotic treatment for or convalescence from a recent illness;
> 4. household contact with a pregnant woman;
> 5. recent exposure to infectious disease;
> 6. breast-feeding;
> 7. a history of allergies, including to penicillin or most other antibiotics; and
> 8. a family history of allergies, adverse reactions, or seizures.[15]

Here, then, twenty years later, is the current ACIP list of recommended vaccines for adults, ages 19 to 65:

2016 ACIP Recommended Adult Immunization Schedule[16]		
Flu	47 doses: 1 yearly	47
Tdap, Td	5 doses: 1 Tdap, then 1 Td every 10 years (plus 1 Tdap for each pregnancy)	5
Chicken pox	2 doses, unless immunocompromised	2
HPV	3 doses: men, 19–22 years; women, 19–26	3

Shingles	1 dose (after age 60)	1
MMR	1–2 doses	1
Pneumo	1–2 doses before age 65, 1 after 65	2
Hepatitis A	2–3 doses	2
Hepatitis B	3 doses	3
Meningococcus	1 dose (or more)	1
Meningococcus B	2–3 doses	2
Hib	1–3 doses	1

This adds up to a total of at least 71 recommended vaccinations, plus another 8 for the extra components of the Tdap, Td, and MMR doses, or 79 altogether, which when added to the 70 recommended for children and adolescents, amounts to a grand total of no fewer than 149 doses of single vaccines and vaccine components from cradle to grave, not even counting the extra doses for seniors over 65, pregnant women, their unborn fetuses, and certain other special indications.

In spite of Dr. Offit's mantra-like reassurances to the contrary, the cumulative effect of so many doses, the ubiquity of autoimmune responses to them, and the common tendency of autoimmune diseases to remain latent and subclinical for months or years all virtually guarantee that anyone adhering faithfully to the CDC schedule, or even a watered-down version of it, is highly likely to develop at least one serious chronic disease, and quite possibly more, to endure and suffer from throughout life, if not actually die from.

To reduce this staggering load that virtually all of us now carry, the most effective way will be simply to end the mandates and make the vaccines purely optional, to offer them to those who want them, and let everyone decide which if any vaccines to give to themselves and their children, a pro-choice policy that is much more in line with what most parents I see are asking for, and what is already happening spontaneously in other countries, given the absence of any genuine public health emergency.

A BETTER MODEL FOR CLINICAL RESEARCH

Providing truly informed consent will also require comprehensive safety and efficacy trials that are designed in a new and radically different way, and are conducted and supervised by an agency that is truly independent of the industry. They could be prospective, with the control groups being given inert placebo, or retrospective, in which case the controls are those much-maligned children and adults who have already chosen not to be vaccinated; and since there are now so many different vaccines to consider, and so many of them contain multiple components, they should include

1. those children and adults who are fully vaccinated, according to current guidelines;
2. those who are partially vaccinated, according to their choices, or those of their parents; and
3. those who choose not to be vaccinated at all.

In other words, nobody is blinded, and everyone receives solely and precisely the level of vaccination and non-vaccination that they choose.

Secondly, the definition of vaccine-related injuries and illnesses needs to be broadened to include both subclinical autoimmune phenomena and overt chronic disease, as well as nonspecific activation and intensification of preexisting conditions and tendencies. This will require lengthening the trial period to several years at least, and the period of active supervision to be made continuous and open-ended, rather than being restricted to specific conditions identified in advance, or giving the investigators broad and exclusive authority to dismiss reports of adverse reactions as "coincidental" without clear guidelines or independent corroboration.

Another important feature will be to include social and psychological parameters, such as intelligence, absenteeism, school and job performance, relationships, temperament, and subjective feelings of contentment, well-being, anxiety, and the like, to give a more complete, well-rounded sense of the health and well-being profile of each individual subject.

Third, the investigators should all be trained clinicians, capable of judging whether or not the reported complaint is vaccine-related, based on attentiveness and sensitivity to the individual patient and the salient circumstances, rather than simply checking off the presence or absence of specific token diagnoses that have already been agreed upon.

Finally, the data should be added to a new database created for that purpose, and the decision to recommend or remove a particular vaccine should continue to be modified in accordance with it.

THE BOTTOM LINE

In light of the evidence, we also need to reexamine the standard argument of the industry and its adherents, so far largely unchallenged, that vaccines are highly cost-effective when compared to the medical and social costs of treating the diseases that they are directed against, and will therefore save the taxpayers large sums of money and restrain the skyrocketing costs of health care to that extent.

As we saw, this claim dates from the Clinton era, with the advent of cost-benefit analysis. In 1992, for example, even before President Clinton took office, Dr. Georges Peter, a prominent pediatrician at Brown University, made the economic case for mandatory vaccination as well as anyone before or since:

> One of the most important medical developments of the 20th Century has been the control of common childhood infectious diseases by the administration of vaccines. With the exception of safe water, no other modality, not even antibiotics, has had such a major effect on mortality reduction and population growth. In the current era of escalating health-care costs, effective childhood vaccines are highly economical and thus represent an efficient use of society's resources. A highly favorable benefit-cost ratio—the ratio of the reduction in the cost of disease to the cost of the vaccination program—has been substantiated by many studies. For example, the MMR program led to a savings of $1.3 billion in disease costs in 1983, with a benefit-cost ratio of 14.4:1; and for each dollar spent on the pertussis vaccine, $2.10 is saved in health-care costs.[17]

Similar cost-benefit analyses were widely invoked to promote most of the second-generation vaccines, notably rotavirus, chicken pox, Hib, and pneumococcus, as well as the most recent ones, even though if not precisely because the corresponding diseases were uncommon, mild and non-life-threatening, in serious decline, or already well-controlled, so that vaccinating against them was unnecessary from a narrowly medical point of view.

But at this point it is or should be obvious that these analyses are woefully incomplete, to say the least, for all of the reasons already cited, namely, that they do not include the costs of caring for

1. the large number of deaths, autoimmune diseases, and brain damage (including autism, ADD and ADHD, GBS, MS, seizures, learning disabilities, etc.) that were not acknowledged as vaccine-related, but have since been shown to be;

2. the even larger volume of common diseases that are merely activated or made worse by vaccines, like all the cases of ear infections, asthma, allergies, etc., representing a nonspecific reaction to the vaccination process *per se,* that were similarly overlooked or denied, and are common enough to be the rule, rather than the exception; and
3. the simultaneous and cumulative effect of the total vaccine load, the piling on of more and more doses, à la Paul Offit, which continues to be ignored to this day.

I hope and expect that the study design I am proposing will demonstrate and ultimately measure the extent of these omissions. But even now, based on what we already know, with so many new vaccines being developed and added to the list all the time, every child being required to receive them, and the entire adult population now next in line, it is clear that Dr. Peter's tidy calculations represent only the uppermost tip of an enormous iceberg, and that, far from being economical, vaccinating everybody against every disease we can think of helps to explain

1. why our health-care system has become so costly;
2. why it devours such an inordinate share of our GDP;
3. why our population is so riddled with chronic disease and scores so poorly on infant mortality and other standard measures of general health.

In short, even in advance of knowing the true figures, it is already clear that our vaccination policy, over and above its inherent unwisdom and the incalculable harm and misery it has caused, is in fact one of the most reckless and wildly expensive medical experiments ever undertaken. To say nothing of correcting the problem, simply alleviating its worst excesses in the short run will be far from easy, because

1. Vaccines and the treatment of chronic disease pervade every aspect of our present health-care system.
2. Treatment is difficult, prolonged, and costly.
3. The system is organized mainly around serving the corporate interests of a hugely wealthy and powerful industry, which not only dictates the agenda of the regulatory agencies, as we saw, but also wields disproportionate influence in Congress.

I have no doubt that it can be done, but it will require a broader vision of what public health and health care are really about, and a common political will with the focus and determination to carry it out, both of which have been in short supply since the Great Depression and the Second World War, and are now in especially short supply, given the ideological polarization of our elected officials, and the paralysis of our government as the inevitable and in some quarters clearly intended result.

LAWS AND EXEMPTIONS

When it comes to enforcing mandates, laws, and exemptions, the present situation is rather more favorable and more amenable to genuine reform than might at first appear, because the ACIP is an arm of the CDC and can only recommend which vaccines should be given and when, whereas the authority both to mandate them and to grant certain exemptions rests ultimately with the individual states, which differ to some extent as to which vaccines are required and what kinds of exemptions are permitted.

Thus the DTaP, IPV, and MMR are mandated in every state, as are the chicken pox (except in South Dakota), the Hib (except in Delaware and Oklahoma), and the hepatitis B (except in Arizona, Montana, and South Dakota), whereas the other three of the second generation (pneumococcus, rotavirus, and influenza) are currently mandated in relatively few states (13, 4, and 3, respectively); and the three most recent ones (meningococcus, hepatitis A, and HPV) in 28, 21, and so far only two states plus the District of Columbia, respectively.[18]

As for exemptions, there are essentially two kinds. All states recognize certain medical exemptions, but these apply only to one vaccine at a time, and only to the very few officially recognized contraindications to each one, as well as having to be renewed on a yearly basis; they were designed to be and have always remained exceedingly difficult to obtain, such that very few individuals can qualify for them.

At least until recently, all states but two also allowed some form of exemption based on a formal religious affiliation, as with the Jehovah's Witnesses, for example; and about twenty allow a "philosophical" exemption based on a deeply held personal belief.[19] On the heels of the Disneyland measles outbreak of 2014, however, California and Vermont have recently enacted new laws eliminating the philosophical or personal-belief exemption; and similar laws are pending at the federal level, as well as in a number of other states.

Furthermore, even where philosophical or personal-belief exemptions remain in force, in most states they stipulate a level of belief that rejects all vaccines on principle and across the board, and thus protect only those willing to identify themselves as deviants in that sense. Above all, they stop well short of a genuinely pro-choice position, which is what many parents say they really want. They do not acknowledge parents' rights of informed consent, or their authority to make intelligent medical decisions for their children, like choosing some vaccines but not others, or specifying when they would like them to be given. In other words, a pro-choice position means simply that the parents are in charge, and that, barring some exceptional circumstance, they should have the say about which if any vaccines they or their children will receive, and when.

In that case, no personal-belief or medical exemption is necessary, since if a sibling has already suffered an adverse reaction, or if the child already suffers from a chronic disease, the parents can decide against the vaccination, just as they might without having to give any reason at all. Conversely, it could easily happen that the physician has good reasons to argue against the vaccine and tries to dissuade the parents, but they are adamant that it be given regardless. In both cases, as more and more vaccines are being added to the list, I am reasonably certain that the pro-choice position will ultimately prevail, although not, I fear, until many more recipients have died or suffered brain damage.

Finally, even when the general public comes around to this belief and finds the way to make such a preference unmistakably clear, it will still be necessary to overcome what might well be called "the vaccine lobby," comprising both the powerful emotional investment of most physicians in vaccination as a premier strategy for fighting disease, and the enormously rich and powerful vested interest of the industry and the CDC in promoting it aggressively to the maximum possible extent. All that has changed is that there are so many vaccines out there, so many aggrieved parents, and so many scandals from within the CDC and the FDA themselves, that the bloom of sanctity surrounding them has been fading away to the point that these corporations and the agencies and physicians who advocate for them can no longer rely quite as smugly as before on the trappings of religion to protect them.

RUNAWAY CAPITALISM IS BAD MEDICINE AND BAD SCIENCE

As we have seen, a number of prominent physicians and scientists, including several former drug industry executives and employees, have already borne witness to the widespread corruption and fraud within the drug industry and the government agencies created to regulate them, involving manipulation and falsification of experimental data, and official assurances to cover them up and deceive the public.

An obvious case in point was the belated admission of Dr. Peter Rost, a former vice president of Pfizer, that all vaccine safety and efficacy studies are funded, designed, and micromanaged by the manufacturers themselves to fabricate whatever results will best promote the virtues and hide the defects of their products, and thus insure and maximize their commercial success.[20]

Even less easily ignored or forgotten are the multifarious and interlocking autism scandals, involving the CDC itself, in which

1. Dr. William Thompson submitted written testimony to Congress that high officials in the CDC ordered him and his colleagues at the agency to bury their own data, which showed a marked increase in autism in young boys who had received the MMR vaccine, and that he continued to do so for many years, until his conscience got the better of him;[21]
2. the CDC denied for many years that thimerosal caused autism, in spite of many studies demonstrating that it did, and hired a Danish investigator to mount faked studies with falsified data to prove that it didn't;[22] and
3. the CDC and the *British Medical Journal* hired a prominent British journalist to ruin the reputation of Dr. Andrew Wakefield, after the latter discovered lesions like those of Crohn's disease in the intestines of several autistic children, and later identified specific antibodies against measles in the ones who had received the MMR vaccine, as a result of which he was fired from his position at a major London hospital, had his article formally retracted, and his license to practice medicine revoked.[23]

Nor is it any secret that Dr. Julie Gerberding, former head of the CDC, recently collected a seven-figure raise from Merck, the company she had ostensibly been hired to regulate, for agreeing to become its vice president in charge of vaccines,[24] a wholly legal and by no means unusual occurrence in the corporate world. Somewhat less widely known are

1. the videos of Brandy Vaughan: a former sales rep for Merck, who after leaving the company has devoted her life, career, and reputation to speaking out on behalf of the vaccine-injured about the pervasive corruption in the drug industry that she witnessed firsthand;[25] and

2. the tell-all book, *Confessions of an Ex-Drug Pusher,* by Gwen Olsen, another sales rep for several drug companies, featuring exclamations like "We're trained to misinform!" and "There's no such thing as a safe drug!"[26]

Even more recently, everybody following the vaccine issue is familiar with the exploits of Dr. Richard Pan, a California pediatrician and state senator, who mostly wrote and has single-handedly championed the infamous bill SB277 abolishing the personal-belief exemption, for which he received a campaign contribution of almost $100,000 as payment from the drug industry, along with other prominent legislators and committee chairmen who were instrumental in approving it.[27]

As we've come to expect, these scandalous revelations are simply business as usual in the drug industry and elsewhere, and although widely known and publicized, they have occasioned little more than mild embarrassment and a few raised eyebrows in the "medical-industrial complex," the mainstream media, and that vast segment of the American medical community and the general public who still rely on the CDC and the journals they sponsor for their vaccine news and information.

I cite them now mainly to point out what we already know, that these instances of corruption are not isolated cases of a few "bad apples," but rather indicative of a deep, systemic problem that is inherent in our current system of interlocking directorates, "revolving doors," and the shared commercial and political interests tying together organized medicine, giant multinational drug companies, and the government agencies ostensibly created to regulate them, just as in other important industries.

In any case, the bad science exemplified by the industry's fraudulent safety studies has already aroused the ire and indignation of some prominent critics from within the medical community itself. One such is Marcia Angell, MD, former editor of the *New England Journal of Medicine,* whose award-winning book *The Truth about the Drug Companies: How They Deceive Us and What to Do about It* provides a tough-minded exposé of the drug industry and its unprecedented dominance over the American medical system, and whose thoughtful and well-researched articles on the same subject resulted in her being fired by the journal; she has since become a professor of social medicine at Harvard Medical School.

Drawing on her long experience as an editor, Dr. Angell catalogues the drug industry's strategies for controlling the conduct of medical research, the education and training of physicians, and the practice of medicine as well, mainly through their readiness and financial capacity to pay handsomely for favorable marketing of their products, precisely the corruption of science that Dr. Rost all but boasted of:

> My 2000 Editorial, "Is Academic Medicine for Sale?" was prompted by a clinical trial of the antidepressant Serzone. The lead author was paid more than half a million dollars in drug-company consulting fees in just one year. But I wouldn't have bothered to write the Editorial if not for the fact that the situation, while extreme, was hardly unique.
>
> Among the many letters I received in response, two were especially pointed. One asked, "Is academic medicine for sale? These days, *everything* is for sale." A second went even further: "Is academic medicine for sale? No. The current owner is very happy with it." The writer didn't feel he had to say who the current owner was.[28]

HEALTH CARE AS A HUMAN RIGHT

What all of these abuses clearly signify is what, again, I think we all know deep down, but have been beguiled or distracted from taking too seriously, let alone losing any sleep over—that health care is a basic human right, not a commodity for sale, or a privilege for the few who can still afford it. In that sense, it is also an allegory for the largely unregulated, "Robber-Baron" style of capitalism under which we presently live, for by no means the first time in our history.

In recent years, Dr. Angell's exposure of the systematic collusion between the drug industry, the academic medical centers and teaching hospitals, the CDC and other government regulatory bodies, and ultimately the medical profession itself, has disillusioned her to the point of repudiating our entire for-profit system, and advocating single-payer health care for all on both ethical and socioeconomic grounds, an avowedly socialist program that was anathema to most physicians for many decades but has since been embraced by the such pillars of the establishment as the Massachusetts Medical Society and a surprisingly large and ever-growing number of practicing physicians:

> Our health-care system is based on the premise that health care is a commodity like VCRs or computers and that it should be distributed according to the ability to pay in the same way that consumer goods are. That's not what health care

should be. Health care is a need; it's not a commodity, and it should be distributed according to need. If you're very sick, you should have a lot of it. If you're not sick, you shouldn't have a lot of it. But this should be seen as a personal, individual need, not as a commodity to be distributed like other marketplace commodities. That is a fundamental mistake in the way this country, and only this country, looks at health care. And that market ideology is what has made the health-care system so dreadful, so bad at what it does.[29]

The way we distribute health care like a market commodity instead of a social good has produced the most expensive, inequitable, and wasteful health system in the world. The United States now spends per capita two and a half times as much on health care as the average for the other OECD countries, while still leaving tens of millions uninsured.[30]

Until we treat health care as a social good instead of a market commodity, there is no way to make it universal, comprehensive, and affordable.[31]

THE NEXT STEP

Although admittedly partial and incomplete, the evidence presented here is already more than enough to raise troubling questions about the safety and efficacy of vaccinations, about the concept of vaccinating as the go-to strategy for fighting epidemic diseases, and about the system of for-profit health care that underlies them. Personally, for all of the reasons I've stated, I have grave doubts about the whole project, as well as the individual vaccines, one by one; and I see no compelling reason for recommending any of them on a mass scale, at least in developed countries with a well-developed public health infrastructure, like our own.

But these questions are admittedly complex and difficult, and much time and energy, diligence, political will, and patience will be required to settle them for good. For the present, until more definitive studies are completed, and given the controversy and polarization that surrounds them, my considered recommendation and heartfelt plea is simply that all routine vaccinations for children and adults alike be made optional—i.e., that they be made available to any who want them, after being fully informed of their risks, and that parents be allowed to pick and choose for their children, without needing an exemption from something that is no longer required.

WHAT I BELIEVE

The idea of eradicating measles or polio has come to seem attractive to us simply because the power of medical science encourages the illusion that it is technically possible; we worship every victory of technology over nature, just as the bullfight ritually celebrates the triumph of human intelligence over the brute beast. That is why we seldom begrudge the drug companies their exorbitant profits and even volunteer the bodies of our own children for their latest experiments. Vaccination is essentially a religious sacrament of our participation in the miracle, an *auto-da-fé* in the name of civilization itself.

But even if, one by one, we could somehow eradicate measles, polio, and all the acute, infectious diseases of mankind, I find it difficult to imagine that we would be any the healthier for it, or that others at least equally serious would not arise to take their places. In particular, trading off the epidemic diseases of the past for the ubiquitous chronic diseases of today seems like a bad bargain medically as well as economically, at least in the industrialized world, where major infectious diseases were already in rapid decline owing to basic improvements in hygiene, sanitation, air and water quality, and so forth. Yet these are the fantasies we are taught to believe in, and the idolatries to which we aspire.

That is why, with all due respect, I have little faith in the sacraments of Merck, GSK, Pfizer, and the rest, preferring the much older truth that the liability to fall ill is deeply rooted in our biological nature, and that the signs and symptoms of illness are expressions of our own life energy, trying our utmost to overcome whatever we are trying to overcome, trying, in short, to heal ourselves. The profoundly irreligious and infinitely hazardous myth that purely technical solutions can be found for illness and all other authentic human problems seems seductively attractive because it bypasses the problem of *healing*, which is a genuine and often laborious miracle, requiring art, caring, and individual attention, and can always *fail* to occur.

We are all authentically at risk of illness and death at every moment: no amount of technology can change that. Yet the quixotic mission of technomedicine is precisely to change that: to stand at all times in the front line against disease, to attack and destroy it whenever and wherever it appears. The discipline I try to be worthy of is far simpler, more wholesome, and more satisfying than that: it consists of nothing more elaborate than giving full attention to the actual lived experience of my patients; recognizing the elements of health and well-being that lie hidden in or inaccessible to them; and offering the relevant science and most suitable medicines to assist and enhance their own innate self-healing capacity. Religion or not, that is the profession I would live by; and though ready and eager to share it, I'll not force it on anyone.

ENDNOTES

CHAPTER ONE

1. Davis, B., et al., *Microbiology,* 2nd ed., Harper, 1973, p. 1346.
2. Ibid.
3. Ibid.
4. Roitt, I., et al., *Immunology,* 5th ed., Mosby, 1998, p. 23 et seq.
5. Ibid., p. 45 et seq.
6. Ibid., p. 121 et seq.
7. Mims, C., et al., *Medical Microbiology,* 2nd ed., Mosby, 1998, p. 63 et seq.
8. Ibid.
9. Ibid., p. 24.
10. Newhouse, M., et al., "A Case-Control Study of Carcinoma of the Ovary," *British Journal of Preventive and Social Medicine* 31:148, 1977.
11. Kölmel, K., et al., "Infections and Melanoma Risk," *Melanoma Research* 9:511, 1999.
12. Wrensch, M., et al., "Does Prior Infection with Varicella-Zoster Virus Influence Risk of Adult Glioma?" *American Journal of Epidemiology* 145:594, 1997.
13. Albonico, H., et al., "Febrile Infectious Childhood Diseases in the History of Cancer Patients and Matched Controls," *Medical Hypotheses* 51:315, 1998.
14. Cf. infra, Chapter 9.
15. Kubota, Y., et al., "Association of Measles and Mumps with Cardiovascular Disease," *Atherosclerosis* 241:682, August 2015.
16. Crosby, A., "Virgin-Soil Epidemics as a Factor in the Aboriginal Depopulation of America," *William and Mary Quarterly* 33:289, 1976.

17. Ibid.
18. Ibid.
19. Conference Exhibit, Graph of United States Measles Cases, *History of Vaccines,* College of Physicians, Philadelphia, 2015.
20. Waaijenborg, S., et al., "Waning of Maternal Antibodies Against Measles, Mumps, Rubella, and Varicella," *Journal of Infectious Diseases* 10:1093, 2013.
21. Schlenker, T., et al., "Measles Herd Immunity," *Journal of the AMA* 267:823, 1992.
22. Davis, op. cit., p. 1418.
23. Buttram, H., "Current Childhood Vaccination Programs: an Overview," *Medical Veritas,* 2008.

CHAPTER TWO

1. Graph of Reported US Measles Cases, 1956–2008, College of Physicians of Philadelphia, historyofvaccines.org, 2015.
2. C. Ma, et al., "Monitoring Progress Toward Elimination of Measles in China," *Bulletin of the World Health Organization* 92:340, May 1, 2015.
3. *Medical World News,* April 14, 1986.
4. Jefferson, T., et al., "Influenza Vaccine: Policy vs. Evidence," *British Medical Journal* 333:912, October 28, 2006.
5. Ratner, H., et al., "The Present State of Polio Vaccines," *Illinois Medical Journal* 118:84 and 118:160, 1969.
6. Humphries, S., and Bystrianyk, R., *Dissolving Illusions: Disease, Vaccines, and the Forgotten History,* published by www.dissolvingillusions.com, 2013, p. 231.
7. Cf. Ratner, op. cit.: "Simply by changes in diagnostic criteria, the number of paralytic cases was predetermined to decrease in 1955–1957, whether or not any vaccine was used."
8. At about the same time, the CDC also tightened its use of the term "epidemic," which before the Salk vaccine had included any outbreak exceeding 20 per 100,000 population; in 1954, the limit was raised to 35 cases per 100,000, which disqualified most of the outbreaks that had been occurring all along from being counted as epidemics.
9. Dauer, C. C., "Reported Whooping Cough Morbidity and Mortality in the United States," *Public Health Report* 58:661, April 23, 1943.
10. "Varicella," American Academy of Pediatrics Brochure, 1996: "Most children who get chicken pox and are otherwise healthy experience no complications

from it. When adults get it, the disease usually lasts longer and is more severe, often developing into pneumonia. Adults are almost 10 times more likely than children under 14 to need hospitalization for the disease and more than 20 times more likely to die from it."

11. Simberkoff, M., et al., "Efficacy of Pneumococcal Vaccine in High-Risk Patients," *New England Journal of Medicine* 315:1318, November 20, 1986.
12. Eskola, J., et al., "Efficacy of a Pneumococcal Conjugate Vaccine against Acute Otitis Media," *New England Journal of Medicine* 344:403, February 8, 2001.
13. Cantekin, E., Letter, *New England Journal of Medicine* 344:1719, May 31, 2001: "The vaccine manufacturer concludes that the new vaccine is effective for prevention. But the data do not support this conclusion. In 1999, the same data were presented to the FDA, which rejected the use of this vaccine in otitis media. But the most interesting results are ecological. In a short time the predicted serotype replacement, as observed with other bacterial vaccines, was realized. With this clear warning sign, it is perilous to push this vaccine."
14. Althouse, B., and Scarpino, S., "Asymptomatic Transmission and the Resurgence of *Bordetella pertussis*," *BMC Medicine* 13:1186, 2015.
15. Martin, S., et al., "Pertactin-Negative *Bordetella pertussis* Strains," *Clinical Infectious Diseases* 60:223, 2015.
16. Long, G., et al., "Acellular Pertussis Vaccination Facilitates *Bordetella parapertussis Infection*," *Proceedings of the Royal Society of Biological Sciences* 10:1098, 2010.
17. Althouse and Scarpino, op. cit.
18. Many of these studies have been collected and summarized in the report, *The Emerging Risks of Live-Virus and Virus-Vectored Vaccines: Vaccine-Strain Virus Infection, Shedding, and Transmission*, by Fisher, B. L., National Vaccine Information Center, 2014, www.NVIC.org, which includes hundreds of references from the scientific literature.
19. Vashisht, N., and Puliyel, J., "Polio Programme: Let Us Declare Victory and Move On," *Indian Journal of Medical Ethics* 9:114, April-June 2012.
20. Greninger, A., et al., "Enterovirus D-68 Strain Associated with Acute Flaccid Myelitis," *Lancet Infectious Diseases* 15:671, June 2015.
21. Goldman, G., and King, P., "Review of the Universal Varicella Vaccination Program," *Vaccine* 13:1680, March 25, 2013: "The mandate was pushed through on the basis of a report by the Antelope Valley Varicella Active Surveillance Program (VASP), based in Los Angeles, which stated that the

vaccine had proven highly effective in reducing the incidence of chicken pox, but neglected to publish or even gather the data for shingles, an omission that led one of the lead authors to resign from the project in protest and publish his own highly critical report at a later date. Corroborating other independent studies, this same investigator found that, although the incidence of varicella was indeed reduced somewhat, there were a significant number of breakthrough cases amounting to nearly 20% of those vaccinated, and that the risk of shingles in a population with a vaccination rate of 50% or more increased substantially within a period of 4–8 years after the shot, with attendant increases in the long-term costs of caring for these patients."

22. Castellsagué, X., et al., "Risk of Newly-Detected Infections and Cervical Abnormalities in Women Seropositive for Naturally-Acquired HPV-16 and HPV-18 Antibodies," *Journal of Infectious Diseases* 10:1093, online version March 8, 2014.
23. Mahmoud, S., "HPV Vaccine May Not Protect against High-Grade Cervical Dysplasias," *Journal of Clinical Oncology* 51:4265, 2013.
24. Cherry, J., "The New Epidemiology of Measles and Rubella," *Hospital Practice,* July 1980, p. 52: "In the booster vaccinees, there was only a modest initial rise in titer, and after a year the level was almost back to where it had been before the booster. In addition we noted a lack of 'take' in 14 other children, most of whom had probably been immunologically stimulated before. In short, the data suggested that another booster dose might not have any lasting effect on waning immunity."
25. National Vaccine Advisory Committee, "The Measles Epidemic," *Journal of the AMA* 266:1547, Sept. 18, 1991.
26. Edmondson, M., et al., "Mild Measles and Secondary Vaccine Failure During a Sustained Outbreak in a Highly-Vaccinated Population," *Journal of the AMA* 263:2467, May 9, 1990.
27. Ibid.
28. Ibid.
29. T. O. vs. Secretary of Health and Human Services, VICP Claim #99-635V.

CHAPTER THREE

1. Dr. Colleen Boyle, in reply to questioning by Rep. Bill Posey (R-FL), House Oversight and Government Reform Committee, November 29, 2012.

2. "ActHiB," Package Insert, Sanofi-Pasteur, 2009, p. 6.
3. Cf. the blogpost "How Are Vaccines Evaluated for Safety?" on the website insidevaccines.com, which publishes these inserts together with detailed and informative commentary, a most valuable resource.
4. "ActHiB," op.cit., p. 6.
5. "Tripedia," Package Insert, Sanofi-Pasteur, 2005, p. 6.
6. Ibid.
7. "Gardasil," Package Insert, Merck, 2015, p. 4.
8. Ibid., summarized in "How Are Vaccines Evaluated for Safety?" op. cit.
9. "Gardasil," Package Insert, op. cit., p. 8.
10. Ibid., p. 4.
11. Ibid., p. 7.
12. Interview with Dr. Peter Rost, in Gardasil documentary, *One More Girl,* posted by Arjun Walia, collective-evolution.com, July 7, 2015.
13. "Adacel," Package Insert, Sanofi-Pasteur, 2012, pp. 2–4.
14. "Fluarix, Quadrivalent" Package Insert, GlaxoSmithKline, 2013, pp. 4–9, 13.
15. "Engerix-B," Package Insert, GlaxoSmithKline, 2012, pp. 6, 8, 9.
16. "Recombivax HB," Package Insert, Merck, 2014, pp. 4, 6, 7.
17. "Hiberix," Package Insert, GlaxoSmithKline, 2012, pp. 4, 5, 8.
18. "PedvaxHiB," Package Insert, Merck, 2010, pp. 1, 6, 7.
19. "Cervarix," Package Insert, GlaxoSmithKline, 2015, pp. 3, 4, 12.
20. "MMR-II," Package Insert, Merck, 2014, pp. 1, 6, 7.
21. "Pneumovax-23," Package Insert, Merck, 2015, pp. 3, 4, 6, 7.
22. "Prevnar," Package Insert, Wyeth-Pfizer, 2009, pp. 1, 15.
23. "Prevnar-13," Package Insert, Wyeth-Pfizer, 2015, pp. 6, 7, 25, 26.
24. "IPOL," Package Insert, Sanofi-Pasteur, 2012, pp. 1, 14.
25. "Rotarix," Package Insert, GlaxoSmithKline, 2014, pp. 5–7, 9.
26. "RotaTeq," Package Insert, Merck, 2014, pp. 4, 5, 9.
27. "Varivax," Package Insert, Merck, 2014, pp. 4, 6, 7.
28. "Zostavax," Package Insert, Merck, 2013, pp. 3–5, 8.
29. World Medical Association, *Ethical Principles for Medical Research Involving Human Subjects,* Helsinki, 1964, amended 2008, ¶32, p. 5.
30. *The Nuremberg Code,* 1947, Wikipedia, ¶1.
31. World Medical Association, op. cit., 24, p. 3.
32. Angell, M., "Drug Companies and Doctors: a Story of Corruption," *New York Review of Books,* January 15, 2009, p. 12.
33. Angell, "Big Pharma, Bad Medicine," *Boston Review,* May 1, 2010, *passim.*

CHAPTER FOUR

1. Mendelsohn, R., *How to Raise a Healthy Child . . . in Spite of Your Doctor,* Contemporary Books, Chicago, 1984, pp. 6–7.
2. Ibid., pp. 210–212, *passim.*
3. Tenpenny, S., *Saying No to Vaccines,* Tenpenny Publishing, Cleveland, 2008, "A Note to Readers," pp. vii-viii, *passim.*
4. Humphries and Bystrianyk, op. cit., Introduction, pp. xii-xiv, *passim.*
5. Bark, T., Letter to Oregon State Senator Ferrioli, posted in *Health Impact News,* October 22, 2015, healthimpactnews.com.
6. Palevsky, L., www.drpalevsky.com, January 2, 2012.
7. Martin, M., and Badalyan, V., "Vaccination Practices among Physicians and Their Children," *Open Journal of Pediatrics* 2:228, 2012.
8. Ibid.
9. Cook, L., "Parents Share Why They Will Never Vaccinate Again," October 11, 2015, www.StopMandatoryVaccination.com.
10. Ibid.
11. Moskowitz, R., "Hidden in Plain Sight: the Rôle of Vaccines in Chronic Disease," *American Journal of Homeopathic Medicine* 98:15, Spring 2005.
12. Moskowitz, "The Case against Immunizations," *Journal of the American Institute of Homeopathy* 76:7, 1983.
13. Moskowitz, 2005, op. cit.
14. Moskowitz, "Vaccination: a Sacrament of Modern Medicine," *Journal of the American Institute of Homeopathy* 84:96, December 1991.
15. Moskowitz, 2005, op. cit.
16. Moskowitz, "Childhood Ear Infections," *Journal of the American Institute of Homeopathy* 87:137, Autumn 1994.
17. Moskowitz, "Hidden in Plain Sight: Vaccines as a Major Risk Factor for Chronic Disease," *American Journal of Homeopathic Medicine* 106:107, Autumn 2013.
18. Moskowitz, 2005, op. cit.
19. Ibid.
20. Moskowitz, 2013, op. cit.

CHAPTER FIVE

1. Wakefield, A., et al., "Measles Vaccine: a Risk Factor for Inflammatory Bowel Disease?" *The Lancet* 345:1071, 1995.

2. Wakefield, et al., "Ileal-Lymphoid Hyperplasia, Nonspecific Colitis, and Pervasive Developmental Disorder in Children," *The Lancet* 351:637, 1998.
3. Cf., for example, D'Euphemia, P., et al., "Abnormal Intestinal Permeability in Children with Autism," *Acta Pædiatrica* 85:1076, 1996; McDonald, T., "The Significance of Ileo-Colonic Lymphoid Nodular Hyperplasia in Children with Autistic Spectrum Disorder," *European Journal of Gastroenterology and Hepatology* 18:569, 2006; and Gonzalez, L., "Gastrointestinal Pathology in Autistic Spectrum Disorders: the Venezuelan Experience," *The Autism File* 32:74, 2009.
4. "List of Autoimmune and Autoimmune-Related Diseases," American Autoimmune-Related Disease Association (AARDA), aarda.org.
5. This list of vaccines and diseases was compiled from the *Physicians' Drug Reference* (*PDR*), 67th ed., 2013.
6. "ACIP Update," *Morbidity and Mortality Weekly Report* 45:22, 1996.
7. Peyriere, H., et al., "Acute Pericarditis after Vaccination against Hepatitis B," *Revue de Médecine Interne* 18:675, 1997. [In French.]
8. Creange, A., et al., "Lumbosacral Acute Demyelinating Neuropathy following Hepatitis B Vaccination," *Autoimmunity* 30:143, 1999.
9. Deisenhammer, F., et al., "Acute Cerebellar Ataxia after Immunisation with Recombinant Hepatitis B Vaccine," *Acta Neurologica Scandinavica* 89:462, 1994.
10. Erbagci, Z., "Childhood Bullous Pemphigoid following Hepatitis B Immunization," *Journal of Dermatology* 29:781, 2002.
11. Ferrande, M., et al., "Lichen Planus following Hepatitis B Vaccination," *British Journal of Dermatology* 139:350, 1998.
12. Fernandez-Funez, A., et al., "Juvenile Dermatomyositis Concomitant with Hepatitis B Vaccination," *Medica Clinica de Barcelona* 111:675, 1998. [In Spanish.]
13. Fraser, P., et al., "Reiter's Syndrome Attributed to Hepatitis B Immunisation," *British Medical Journal* 309:1315, 1994.
14. Fried, M., et al., "Uveitis after Hepatitis B Vaccination," *The Lancet* 8559:631, 1987.
15. Granel, B., et al., "Occlusion of Central Retinal Vein after Vaccination against Viral Hepatitis B with Recombinant Vaccines," 4 cases, *Presse Medicale* 26:62, 1997. [In French.]
16. Hanzawa, S., et al., "A Case of Membranoproliferative Glomerulonephritis Associated with Hepatitis B Vaccine," *Nippon Jinzo Gakkai Shi* 22:41, 1980. [In Japanese.]

17. Halsey, N., et al., "Hepatitis B Vaccine and CNS Demyelinating Diseases," *Pediatric Infectious Diseases* 18:23, 1999.
18. Heinzlef, O., et al., "Acute Aseptic Meningitis after Hepatitis B Vaccination," *Presse Medicale* 26:328, 1997. [In French.]
19. Hutteroth, T., et al., "Aluminum Hydroxide Granuloma following Hepatitis B Vaccination, *Deutsche Medizinische Wochenschrift* 115:476, 1990. [In German.]
20. DeLernia, V., et al., "Erythema Multiforme following Hepatitis B Vaccine," *Pediatric Dermatology* 11:363, 1994.
21. Macario, F., et al., "Nephrotic Syndrome after Recombinant Hepatitis B Vaccine," *Clinical Nephrology* 43:349, 1995.
22. Mathieu, E., et al., "Cryoglobulinemia after Hepatitis B Vaccination," *New England Journal of Medicine* 335:355, 1996.
23. Pope, J., et al., "The Development of Rheumatoid Arthritis after Recombinant Hepatitis B vaccination," *Journal of Rheumatology* 25:1687, 1998.
24. Toft, J., et al., "Subacute Thyroiditis after Hepatitis B Vaccination," *Endocrine Journal* 45:135, February 1998.
25. Matsuura, E., et al., "Is Atherosclerosis an Autoimmune Disease?" *BMC Medicine* 12:47, 2014.
26. Shoenfeld, Y., et al., eds., *Vaccines and Autoimmunity,* WILEY Blackwell, 2015, Introduction, p. 1.
27. Ibid., pp. 1, 2, *passim.*
28. Ibid., pp. 2–4, *passim.*
29. "Estimated Prevalence of Autism and Other Developmental Disabilities," *National Health Statistics Reports,* National Center for Health Statistics, Nov. 13, 2015, CDC, cdc.gov.
30. Gies, W., "Some objections to the use of alum baking powder," *Journal of the AMA* 57:816, 1911, cited in Tomljenovic, L., and Shaw, C., "Answers to Common Misconceptions Regarding the Toxicity of Aluminum Adjuvants in Vaccines," in *Vaccines and Autoimmunity,* op. cit., Chapter 4.
31. Cf. Shaw, C., and Petrik, M., "Aluminum Hydroxide Injections Lead to Motor Deficits and Motor Neuron Degeneration," *Journal of Inorganic Biochemistry* 103:1555, 2009, cited in *Vaccines and Autoimmunity,* op. cit., Chapter 4.
32. Tomljenovic, L., "Aluminum and Alzheimer's Disease: after a Century of Controversy, Is There a Plausible Link?" *Journal of Alzheimer's Disease* 23:567, 2011, cited in *Vaccines and Auto-immunity,* op. cit., Chapter 4.

33. Cf., for example, Seneff, S., "Empirical Data Confirm Autism Symptoms Related to Aluminum and Acetaminophen Exposure," *Entropy* 14:2227, 2012, cited in *Vaccines and Autoimmunity,* op. cit., Chapter 4.
34. Shoenfeld, Y., and Agmon-Levin, N., "ASIA: Autoimmune/Inflammatory Syndrome Induced by Adjuvants," *Journal of Autoimmunity* 36:4, 2011.
35. Shaw and Petrik, op. cit., 2009.
36. Tomljenovic and Shaw, *Vaccines and Autoimmunity,* op. cit., Chapter 4, p. 47.
37. Offit, P., and Jew, R., "Addressing Parents' Concerns: Do Vaccines Contain Harmful Preservatives, Adjuvants, Additives, or Residuals?" *Pediatrics* 112:1394, 2003.
38. Tomljenovic and Shaw, *Vaccines and Immunity,* op. cit., Chapter 4, p. 45.

CHAPTER SIX

1. "Developmental Disabilities," "ADHD," and "Autism-Spectrum Disorder," CDC, cdc.gov.
2. Unpublished letter to the author.
3. Moskowitz, R., "Hidden in Plain Sight: the Rôle of Vaccines in Chronic Disease," *American Journal of Homeopathic Medicine* 98:15, Spring 2005.
4. Coulter, H., and Fisher, B. L., *DPT: a Shot in the Dark,* Harcourt Brace Jovanovich, 1985.
5. Stewart, G., "Vaccination against Whooping-Cough: Efficacy vs. Risks," *Lancet* 309:234, Jan. 28, 1977.
6. Ibid.
7. Ibid.
8. Ibid.
9. Ibid.
10. Vide infra, Chapter 12.
11. US Dept. of Health and Human Services, Health Resources and Services Administration (HRSA), "VICP Data and Statistics," updated October 2015, p. 5.
12. Kessler, D., "Introducing MEDWatch: a New Approach to Reporting Medication and Device Adverse Effects," *Journal of the AMA* 269:2765, June 2, 1993.
13. Mortimer, E., et al., "The Risk of Seizures and Encephalopathy after Immunization with the DPT Vaccine," *Journal of the AMA* 263:1641, March 23, 1990.

14. Cherry, J., "Pertussis Vaccine Encephalopathy: It's Time to Recognize It as the Myth That It Is," *Journal of the AMA* 263:1679, March 23, 1990.
15. "Vaccine Side Effects, Adverse Reactions, Contraindications & Precautions," Advisory Committee on Immunization Practices, *Morbidity and Mortality Weekly Report* 45:22, September 1996.
16. Kanner, L., "Autistic Disturbances of Affective Contact," *Nervous Child* 2:217, 1943.
17. Wakefield, A., et al., "Measles Vaccine: a Risk Factor for Inflammatory Bowel Disease?" *Lancet* 345:1071, 1995.
18. Ibid.
19. Wakefield, et al., "Ileal Lymphoid-Nodular Hyperplasia, Non-Specific Colitis, and Pervasive Developmental Disorder in Children," *Lancet* 351:637, 1998.
20. Wakefield, "Autism and Childhood Vaccines," Testimony before Congressional Oversight Committee on Autism and Immunization, C-Span, April 6, 2000.
21. Cf., for example, Taylor, B., et al., "Autism and MMR Vaccine: No Epidemiological Evidence for a Causal Association," *Lancet* 353:2026, 1999.
22. Deer, B., "How the Case against the MMR Was Fixed," "How the Vaccine Crisis Was Meant to Make Money," "*The Lancet*'s Two Days to Bury Bad News," and "Pathology Reports Solve the 'New Bowel Disease' Riddle," *British Medical Journal,* January 5, 11, 19, and November 9, 2011.
23. Ibid.
24. Horton, R., "A Statement by the Editors," *Lancet* 363:820, 2004.
25. Ibid.
26. Ibid.
27. "British Medical Council Bars Doctor Who Linked Vaccine with Autism," *New York Times,* May 24, 2010.
28. "Documents Emerge Proving Dr. Walker-Smith Innocent," NaturalNews.com, January 26, 2011, and "MMR Doctor Wins High Court Appeal," *BBC News,* March 7, 2012.
29. Cf., for example, Horvath, K., et al., "Gastrointestinal Abnormalities in Children with Autistic Disorder," *Journal of Pediatrics* 135:559, 1999; Ashwood, P., et al., "Intestinal Lymphocyte Populations in Children with Regressive Autism," *Journal of Clinical Immunology* 23:504, 2003; Singh, V., and Jensen, R., "Elevated Levels of Measles Antibodies in Children with Autism," *Pediatric Neurology* 28:1, 2003; and Galiatsatos, P., et al., "Autistic Enterocolitis: Fact or Fiction?" *Canadian Journal of Gastroenterology* 23:95, 2009.

30. Wakefield, "MMR, Enterocolitis, and Autism," Lecture, NVIC International Conference, Washington, November 2002.
31. Ibid.
32. Cf., for example, Megson, M., "Genetics, Vaccine Injury, and Getting Well," Lecture, NVIC Annual Conference, 2002.
33. Attkisson, S., "Family to Receive $1,500,000 in First-Ever Vaccine Court Award," *CBS News,* September 10, 2010.
34. "Identified Prevalence of Autism Spectrum Disorder," CDC Data and Statistics, ASD home page, cdc.gov.
35. Healy, B., Interview with Sharyl Attkisson, *CBS News,* May 12, 2008.
36. *DSM-V, Diagnostic and Statistical Manual of Mental Disorders,* 5th ed., American Psychiatric Association, 2013, Section II, "Diagnostic Criteria and Codes, Neurodevelopmental Disorders."
37. Ibid.
38. ASD home page, CDC, cdc.gov.
39. Ibid.
40. Kennedy, Robert F., Jr., ed., *Thimerosal: Let the Science Speak,* Skyhorse, New York, 2014.
41. Gallagher, C., et al., "Hepatitis B Vaccination of Male Neonates and Autism," *Annals of Epidemiology* 19:651, 2009.
42. Goth, S., et al., "Uncoupling of ATP-Mediated Calcium Signaling and Dysregulated Interleukin-6 Secretion in Dendritic Cells by Nanomolar Thimerosal," *Environmental Health Perspectives* 114:1083, 2006.
43. Burbacher, T., "Comparison of Blood and Brain Mercury Levels in Infant Monkeys Exposed to Methylmercury or Vaccines Containing Thimerosal," *Environmental Health Perspectives* 113:1015, 2005.
44. Waly, M., et al., "Activation of Methionine Synthetase by Insulin-Like Growth Factor 1 and Dopamine: a Target for Neurodevelopmental Toxins and Thimerosal," *Molecular Psychiatry* 9:358, 2004 (online).
45. De Soto, M., et al., "Blood Levels of Mercury Are Related to Diagnosis of Autism," *Journal of Child Neurology* 22:1308, 2007.
46. Geier, D., and Geier, M., "A Case Series of Children with Apparent Mercury Toxic Encephalopathies Manifesting with Clinical Symptoms of Regressive Autistic Disorder," *Journal of Toxicology and Environmental Health* 70:837, 2007.
47. Cheuk, D., and Wong, V., "Attention-Deficit Hyperactivity Disorder and Blood Mercury Level: a Case-Control Study of Chinese Children," *Neuropediatrics* 37:234, 2006.

48. Natafa, R., et al., "Porphyrinuria in Childhood Autistic Disorder: Implications for Environmental Toxicity," *Toxicology and Applied Phrmacology* 214:99, 2006.
49. Ratajczak, H., "Theoretical Aspects of Autism: Causes—a Review," *Journal of Immunotoxicology* 8:68, 2011.
50. Herbert, M., "Autism: a Brain Disorder, or a Disorder That Affects the Brain?" *Clinical Neuropsychiatry* 2:354, 2005.
51. Werner, E., and Dawson, G., "Validation of the Phenomenon of Autistic Regression Using Home Videotapes," *Archives of General Psychiatry* 62:889, 2005.
52. Poling, J., et al., "Developmental Regression and Mitochondrial Dysfunction in a Child with Autism," *Journal of Child Neurology* 21:170, 2006.
53. Shaw, C., "Aluminum Adjuvant Linked to Gulf War Illness Induces Motor Neuron Death in Mice," *Neuromolecular Medicine* 9:83, 2007.
54. Blaxill, M., et al., "The Changing Prevalence of Autism in California," *Journal of Autism and Developmental Disorders* 33:223, 2003.
55. Gargus, J., and Imtiaz, F., "Mitochondrial Energy-Deficient Endophenotype in Autism," *American Journal of Biochemistry and Biotechnology* 4:198, 2008.
56. Press Release, "Statement of William W. Thompson, Ph. D., Regarding the 2004 Article Examining the Possibility of a Relationship between the MMR Vaccine and Autism," August 27, 2014, Morgan Verkamp LLC.
57. Written Statement of Dr. Thompson, submitted to Rep. William Posey (R-FL), and read by him *verbatim* on the House floor: excerpts reported by Sharyl Attkisson, *CBS News,* July 29, 2015, and by Thinking Moms' Revolution, posted August 4, 2015, thinkingmomsrevolution.com.
58. Madsen, K., Thorsen, P., et al., "Thimerosal and the Occurrence of Autism: Negative Ecological Evidence from a Danish Population-Based Study," *Pediatrics* 112:604, 2008.
59. Kennedy, Robert F. Jr., "Central Figure in CDC Vaccine Coverup Absconds with $2 Million," *Huffington Post,* May 11, 2010.
60. Madsen, Thorsen, et al., op. cit.
61. Kennedy, R. F. Jr., *Huffington Post,* op. cit.

CHAPTER SEVEN

1. Steinschneider, A., "Prolonged Apnea and the Sudden Infant Death Syndrome," *Pediatrics* 50:64, 1972.

2. Cf., for example, Southall, D., "The Role of Apnea in the Sudden Infant Death Syndrome," *Pediatrics* 81:73, 1988.
3. Miller, N., and Goldman, G., "Infant Mortality Rates Regressed Against the Number of Vaccine Doses Routinely Given," *Human and Experimental Toxicology* online, May 4, 2011; Press Release, Think Twice Global Vaccine Institute, www.thinktwice.com.
4. CDC, "About SUID and SIDS," cdc.gov.
5. CDC, "SUID and SIDS," Vital Statistics Data, "Linked Birth-Infant Death Files," cdc.gov.
6. Ibid.
7. Cf., for example, Jeffery, H., et al., "Why the Prone Position Is a Risk Factor for Sudden Infant Death Syndrome," *Pediatrics* 104:263, 1999.
8. Bernier, R., et al., "DTP Vaccination and Sudden Infant Deaths in Tennessee," *Journal of Pediatrics* 101:419, 1982.
9. Torch, W., "DPT Immunization: a Potential Cause of Sudden Infant Death Syndrome," *Neurology* 32:169, 1982.
10. Ibid.
11. Noble, G., et al., "Acellular and Whole-Cell Pertussis Vaccines in Japan," *Journal of the AMA* 257:1351, 1987.
12. Cherry, J., et al., "Report of Task Force on Pertussis and Pertussis Immunization," Supplement, *Pediatrics* 81:939, 1988.
13. Scheibner, V., *Vaccination: a Medical Assault on the Immune System,* New Atlantean Press, 1993, pp. xiii-xv, *passim.*
14. "Hepatitis B Vaccine," Special Report, *The Vaccine Reaction,* National Vaccine Information Center, September 1998.
15. "Gardasil Vaccine: One More Girl Dead," *Health Impact News,* August 11, 2014, healthimpactnews.com.
16. "Girl with Sore Throat Gets HPV Vaccine, Dies Hours Later," *Fox 4 News,* Kansas City, August 8, 2014, fox4kc.com.
17. "In Loving Memory of Otto Geiger," June 1, 2015, www.gofundme.com.
18. Farber, C., "A Family Destroyed: Six-Month-Old Dies after Clinic Injects Baby with 13 Vaccines at Once Without Informed Consent," *Natural News,* May 19, 2015, naturalnews.com.
19. Ursino, A., "California Infant Dies after 8 Vaccines, Family Gets Him Back from Hospital Cremated," *VacTruth,* February 26, 2015, vactruth.com.
20. England, C., "Vaccine Bombshell: Leaked Confidential Document Exposes 36 Infants Dead after This Vaccine," *VacTruth,* December 16, 2012, vactruth.com.

21. "Vaccine Proven to Cause Sudden Death in Children," *Child Health Safety,* January 13, 2015, childhealthsafety.wordpress.com.
22. "Personal Stories of Vaccine Injury and Death," Think Twice Global Vaccine Institute, www.thinktwice.com.
23. Ibid.
24. Ibid.
25. Ibid.
26. Ibid.
27. Ibid.
28. Ibid.
29. Ibid.
30. Ibid.
31. Ibid.
32. Offit, P., et al., "Addressing Parents' Concerns: Do Multiple Vaccines Overwhelm or Weaken the Infant's Immune System?" *Pediatrics* 109:124, 2002.
33. Javier Cardenal Taján, "GlaxoSmithKline Found Guilty in Deaths of 14 Babies in Vaccine Trials in Argentina," *Buenos Aires Herald,* January 3, 2012, reported in *Health Impact News,* healthimpactnews.com.
34. Mario Lamo-Jiménez, "Breaking News: Vaccine Tragedy in Mexico," SaneVax, Inc., May 11, 2015, sanevax.org.
35. Kumar, N., "Controversial Vaccine Studies: Why Is the Bill & Melinda Gates Foundation Under Fire in India?" *Economic Times of India,* August 30, 2014.
36. Ibid.
37. *Orlando Sentinel,* August 28, 2004, p. 1.
38. "'Shaken Baby' Conviction Overturned," *British Medical Journal* 328:719, 2004.
39. Ibid.
40. Innis, M., "Shaken-Baby Syndrome—Shaken," *VacTruth,* October 27, 2015, vactruth.com.
41. "Vaccine Injuries and Death Payments," U.S. Department of Justice Report, March 5, 2015, *Health Impact News,* healthimpactnews.com.
42. Ibid.
43. Barbara Loe Fisher, "In Memoriam: Infant Death and Vaccination," *The Vaccine Reaction,* NVIC, May 25, 2011.

CHAPTER EIGHT

1. Holland, M., "Unanswered Questions from the Vaccine Injury Compensation Program: a Review of Compensated Cases of Vaccine-Induced Brain Injury," *Pace Environmental Law Review* 28:480, March 28, 2011.
2. Iskander, J., et al., "Vaccine Safety Post-Marketing Surveillance: the Vaccine Adverse Event Reporting System," CDC, cdc.gov, 2004, p. 2.
3. Ibid., "Evaluating Side Effects After Vaccination: Temporal vs. Causal Associations," Table 1, p. 3
4. "Table of Reportable Events Following Vaccination," cdc.gov/vaccines, 2008.
5. "Vaccine Injury Table," Health Resources and Services Administration, Department of Health and Human Services, hrsa.gov, June 23, 2015.
6. Piper-Terry, M., "The Trouble with VAERS," *ADHD/ASD Recovery*, Shawn Siegel, co-host, YouTube, March 16, 2014.
7. Belkin, M., "Hepatitis B," Think Twice Global Vaccine Institute, think-twice.com, based on Congressional testimony, May 18, 1999, United States Government Printing Office, p. 67 et seq., *passim.*
8. "Guerrilla RN," communitybabycenter.com, October 22, 2015, *passim.*
9. Holland, M., et al., op. cit., Part I, p. 484.
10. Ibid., pp. 485–489, *passim.*
11. Holland, M., and Krakow, R., "The Right to Legal Redress," in *The Vaccine Epidemic,* Holland, M., and Habakus, L., eds., Skyhorse, 2011, pp. 39–40, *passim.*
12. Satcher, D., Surgeon-General of the United States, Congressional testimony, August 3, 1999, cited by Tenpenny, S., "A Doctor's View of Vaccines and the Public Health," in *Vaccine Epidemic,* op. cit., p. 184.
13. "Petitions Filed, Compensated, and Dismissed," National Vaccine Injury Compensation Program, Health Resources and Services Administration, HHS, hrsa.gov, p. 5.
14. Ibid., p. 1, "Data and Statistics."
15. Rohde, W., *The Vaccine Court,* Skyhorse, New York, 2014, pp. 92–93.
16. T. O. v. Secretary of HHS, #99-635V.
17. Ibid.
18. L. K. v. Secretary of HHS, #99-624V.
19. J. O. v. Secretary of HHS, #99-636V.
20. Fisher, B., "Vaccine Injury Compensation: Government's Broken Social Contract with Parents," *The Vaccine Reaction,* November 2, 2015, nvic.org.

CHAPTER NINE

1. Miller, N., and Goldman, G., "Infant Mortality Rates Regressed against the Number of Vaccine Doses Routinely Given," *Human Experimental Toxicology* 30:1420, 2011.
2. Ibid.
3. Ibid.
4. Goldman, G., and Miller, N., "Relative Trends in Hospitalizations and Mortality among Infants by the Number of Vaccine Doses and Age, Based on the VAERS Reporting System, 1990–2010," *Human Experimental Toxicology* 31:1012, 2012.
5. Glanz, J., et al., "A Population-Based Cohort Study of Under-Vaccination in 8 Managed Care Organizations across the United States," *JAMA Pediatrics* 167:284, 2013.
6. Olmsted, D., "The Amish All Over Again," *Age of Autism*, May 12, 2012, ageofautism.com.
7. Attkisson, S., "Where Are the Autistic Amish?" sharylattkisson.com, July 20, 2014.
8. Claridge, S., "Unvaccinated Children Are Healthier," *Investigate before You Vaccinate*, vaccineinjury.info, 2005.
9. Ibid.
10. Odent, M., et al., "Pertussis Vaccination and Asthma: Is There a Link?" Letter, *JAMA* 272:592, 1994.
11. Kemp, T., et al., "Is Infant Immunization a Risk Factor for Childhood Asthma or Allergy?" *Epidemiology* 8:678, 1997.
12. Sun, Y., et al., "Risk of Febrile Seizures and Epilepsy after Vaccination with Diphtheria, Tetanus, Acellular Pertussis, Inactivated Poliovirus, and *Hæmophilus influenzæ* Type B," *JAMA* 307:823, 2012.
13. Ibid.
14. Ibid.
15. Ibid.
16. Von Spiczak, S., et al., "A Retrospective, Population-Based Study of Seizures Related to Childhood Vaccinations," *Epilepsia* 52:1506, 2011.
17. Classen, J., and Classen, D., "Clustering of Cases of IDDM Occurring 3 Years after HiB Immunization Support a Causal Relationship," *Autoimmunity* 35:247, 2002.
18. Ibid.
19. Ibid.

20. Classen and Classen, "Clustering of Cases of Type 1 Diabetes 2–4 Years after Vaccination," *Journal of Pediatric Endocrinology* 16:495, 2003.
21. Classen, J., "Clustering of Cases of IDDM 2–4 Years after Hep B Vaccination Is Consistent with Clustering after Infections and Progression to IDDM in Autoantibody-Positive Individuals," *Open Pediatric Medical Journal* 2:1, 2008.
22. Ibid.
23. Ibid.
24. Ibid.
25. Classen, "Risk of Vaccine-Induced Diabetes in Children with a Family History of Type 1 Diabetes," *Open Pediatric Medical Journal* 2:7, 2008.
26. Ibid.
27. Ibid.
28. Ibid.
29. Rinaldi, M., et al., "ITP: an Autoimmune Cross-Link between Infections and Vaccines," *Lupus* 6:554, 2014.
30. Bertuola, F., et al., "Association between Drug and Vaccine Use and Acute ITP in Childhood: a Case Control Study in Italy," *Drug Safety* 33:65, 2010.
31. Nagasaki, J., et al., "Post-Influenza Vaccine ITP in Three Elderly Patients," *Case Reports in Hematology* 2016:1, 2016.
32. O'Leary, S., et al., "The Risk of ITP after Vaccination in Children and Adolescents," *Pediatrics* 129:248, 2012.
33. Ibid.
34. Ibid.
35. Ibid.
36. Pourcyrous, M., et al., "Primary Immunization of Premature Infants with Gestational Age Less than 35 Weeks," *Journal of Pediatrics* 151:167, 2007.
37. Ibid.
38. Ibid.
39. Ibid.
40. Ibid.
41. Flatz-Jequier, A., et al., "Recurrence of Cardiorespiratory Events Following Repeat DTaP-Based Combined Immunization in Very Low Birth-Weight Premature Infants," *Journal of Pediatrics* 153:429, 2008.
42. Sen, S., et al., "Adverse Events Following Vaccination in Premature Infants," *Acta Pædiatrica* 90:916, 2001.
43. Ibid.
44. Ibid.

CHAPTER TEN

1. Hornig, M., et al., "Neurotoxic Effects of Post-Natal Thimerosal Are Mouse-Strain Dependent," *Molecular Psychiatry* 9:833, 2004.
2. Goth, S., et al., "Uncoupling of ATP-Mediated Calcium Signaling and Dysregulated Interleukin-6 Secretion in Dendritic Cells by Nanomolar Thimerosal," *Environmental Health Perspectives* 114:1083, July 2006.
3. Clarke, D., and Sokoloff L., "Circulation and Energy Metabolism of the Brain," in *Basic Neurochemistry*, Siegel, G., ed., Lippincott, 1999., pp. 637–669.
4. Sharpe, M., et al., "Thimerosal-Derived Ethylmercury Is a Mitochondrial Toxin in Human Astrocytes," *Journal of Toxicology* 2012:373678, 2012 (online).
5. Olczak, M., et al., "Lasting Neuropathological Changes in the Rat Brain after Neonatal Administration of Thimerosal," *Folia Neuropathologica* 48:258, 2010.
6. Duszczyk-Budathoki, M., et al., "Administration of Thimerosal to Infant Rats Increases Overflow of Glutamate and Aspartate in the Prefrontal Cortex," *Neurochemistry Research* 37:436, 2012.
7. Dingledine, R., and McBain, C., "Glutamate and Aspartate Are the Major Excitatory Neurotransmitters in the Brain," in Siegel, op. cit, pp.315–333.
8. Tomljenovic, L., "Aluminum and Alzheimer's Disease," *Journal of Alzheimer's Disease* 23:567, 2011.
9. Klatzo, I., et al., "Experimental Production of Neurofibrillary Degeneration," *Neuropathology and Experimental Neurology* 24:187, 1965.
10. Walton, J., "Functional Impairment in Aged Rats Exposed to Human Range Dietary Aluminum Equivalents," *Neurotoxicology* 30:182, 2009.
11. Yokel, R., et al., "Aluminum Bioavailability from Basic Sodium Aluminum Phosphate, an Approved Food Additive," *Food Chemistry and Toxicology* 46:2261, 2009.
12. Yokel, R.A., and McNamara, P., "Aluminum Toxicokinetics: an Updated Review," *Pharmacology and Toxicology* 88:159, 2001.
13. Exley, C., "Aluminium and Medicine," in *Molecular and Supramolecular Bio-Inorganic Chemistry*, Merce, A., et al., eds., Nova Biomedical Books, 2009, pp. 45–68.
14. Flarend, R., et al., "*In vivo* Absorption of Aluminum-Containing Vaccine Adjuvants Using Aluminum-26," *Vaccine* 15:1314, 1997.
15. Gherardi, R., et al., "Central Nervous System Disease in Patients with Macrophagic Myofascitis," *Brain* 124:974, 2001.

16. Ibid.
17. Eickhoff, T., and Myers, M., "Aluminum in Vaccines," Workshop Summary, Supplement 3, *Vaccine* 20:S1.
18. Gherardi, "Lessons from Macrophagic Myofasciitis: Towards Definition of a Vaccine Adjuvant-Related Syndrome," *Revue Neurologique* (Paris) 159:162, 2003.
19. Zinka, B., et al., "Unexplained Cases of Sudden Infant Death Shortly after Hexavalent Vaccination," *Vaccine* 24:5779, 2006.
20. Ibid.
21. Ibid.
22. Ibid.
23. Lukiw, W., and Bazan, N., "Neuroinflammatory Signaling Upregulation in Alzheimer's Disease," *Neurochemical Research* 25:1173, 2000.
24. Pardo, C., et al., "Immunity, Neuroglia, and Neuroinflammation in Autism," *International Review of Psychiatry* 17:485, 2005.
25. Exley, C., et al., "Elevated Urinary Excretion of Aluminium and Iron in Multiple Sclerosis," *Multiple Sclerosis* 12:533, 2006.
26. Shirabe, T., et al., "Autopsy Case of Aluminum Encephalopathy," *Neuropathology* 22:206, 2002.
27. Exley, C., *Aluminium and Alzheimer's Disease,* Elsevier, 2001.
28. Blaylock, R., and Strunecka, A., "Immune Glutamatergic Dysfunction as a Central Mechanism of Autism Spectrum Disorders," *Current Medicinal Chemistry* 16:157, 2009.
29. Exley, et al., *Multiple Sclerosis,* op. cit., 2006.
30. Flendrig, J., et al., "Aluminum Intoxication: the Cause of Dialysis Dementia?" *Proceedings of the European Dialysis and Transplantation Association* 13:355, 1976.
31. Mailloux, R., et al., "Aluminum-Induced Mitochondrial Dysfunction Leads to Lipid Accumulation in Hepatocytes," *Cell Physiology and Biochemistry* 20:627, 2007.
32. Natafa, R., et al., "Porphyrinuria in Childhood Autistic Disorder: Implications for Environmental Toxicity," *Toxicology and Applied Phrmacology* 214:99, July 15, 2006.
33. CDC 2010 Child & Adolescent Vaccination Schedule, www.cdc.gov/vaccines.
34. Haddad, S., et al., "Characterization of Age-Related Changes in Body and Organ Weights from Birth to Adolescence in Humans," *Journal of Toxicology and Environmental Health* 64:453, 2001.
35. Ibid.

36. Tomljenovic, L., and Shaw, C., "Aluminum Vaccine Adjuvants: Are They Safe?" *Current Medicinal Chemistry* 18:2630, 2011.
37. Ibid.
38. Shoenfeld, Y., et al., eds., *Vaccines & Autoimmunity,* WILEY Blackwell, 2015, Introduction, pp. 2–4, *passim.*
39. Perricone, C., et al., "Measles, Mumps, and Rubella: a Triad to Autoimmunity," in *Vaccines & Autoimmunity,* op. cit., pp. 129–130.
40. Ibid., p. 132.
41. Smyk, D., et al., "Hepatitis B Vaccination and Autoimmunity," in *Vaccines & Autoimmunity,* op. cit., pp. 147–155.
42. Tomljenovic, L., and Shaw, C., "Adverse Reactions to Human Papilloma Virus Vaccines," in *Vaccines & Autoimmunity,* op. cit., pp. 163–174.
43. Ibid., pp. 165–166.
44. Jara, L., et al., "Influenza Vaccine and Autoimmune Diseases," in *Vaccines & Autoimmunity,* op. cit., p. 180.
45. Borrella, E., et al., "Pneumococcal Vaccines and Autoimmune Phenomena," in *Vaccines & Autoimmunity,* op. cit., p. 194.
46. Blank, M., and Cruz-Tapias, P., "Antiphospholipid Syndrome and Vaccines," in *Vaccines & Autoimmunity,* op. cit., pp. 141–145.
47. "What Is Autoimmunity?" Autoimmune Disease Research Center, Johns Hopkins Medical Institutions, autimmune.pathology.jhmi.edu, 2001.
48. HogenEsch, H., et al., "Vaccine-Induced Autoimmunity in the Dog," *Advances in Veterinary Medicine* 41:733, 1999.
49. Ibid.
50. Moghaddam, A., et al., "A Potential Mechanism for Hypersensitivity Caused by Formalin-Inactivated Vaccines," *Nature Medicine* 12:996, 2006.
51. Azadi, S., et al., "Divergent Immunological Responses Following Glutaraldehyde Exposure," *Toxicology & Applied Pharmacology* 197:1, 2004.
52. Mubhoff, U., "2-Phenoxyethanol: A Neurotoxicant? A Reply," Letter to the Editor, *Archives of Toxicology* 74:284, 2000.
53. Palevsky, L., "Aluminum and Vaccine Ingredients: What Do We Know? What Don't We Know?" *International Medical Council on Vaccination*, 2009.
54. Greenwood, J., et al., "The Effect of Bile Salts on the Permeability of the Rat Blood-Brain Barrier," *Journal of Cerebral Blood Flow Metabolism* 11:644, 1991.
55. Shoenfeld et al., Introduction, *Vaccines & Autoimmunity,* op. cit., Table 1.2, pp. 4–5
56. Ibid.

57. Palevsky, L., Interview, *The Pet Whisperer,* thepetwhisperer.com, January 3, 2012.
58. Horwin, M., "SV40: a Cancer-Causing Monkey Virus From FDA-Approved Vaccines," *Albany Law Journal of Science & Technology* 13:721, 2003.
59. Ibid.
60. Shoenfeld, et al., Introduction, *Vaccines & Autoimmunity,* op. cit., pp. 4–5.
61. Krause, P., "Adventitious Agents and Vaccines," FDA, National Center for Biotechnology Information, ncbi.nlm.nih.gov, 2001.
62. "Beta-Propiolactone," Wikipedia, wikipedia.org.
63. Shoenfeld, et al., Introduction, *Vaccines & Autoimmunity,* op. cit., Table 1.2, pp. 4–5.

CHAPTER ELEVEN

1. Cherry, J., et al., "Report of Task Force on Pertussis and Pertussis Immunization," Supplement, *Pediatrics* 81:939, 1988.
2. "Ingredients: Infanrix (DTaP GlaxoSmithKline)," 2011, vaccines.ProCon.org. The other DTaP vaccines, Daptacel and Tripedia (Sanofi-Pasteur), contain only slightly different versions of the same or similar ingredients. In such cases, in the interest of simplicity I have selected one product to represent them all.
3. Dauer, C. C., "Reported Whooping Cough Morbidity and Mortality in the United States," *Public Health Report* 58:661, April 23, 1943.
4. Stewart, G., "Vaccination against Whooping-Cough: Efficacy vs. Risks," *Lancet* 309:234, Jan. 28, 1977.
5. Stewart, "Whooping Cough in Relation to Other Childhood Infections in the UK," *Journal of Epidemiology and Community Health* 35:145, 1981.
6. "Pertussis Cases, Year by Year, 1922–2014," CDC, cdc.gov.
7. Martin, S., et al., "Pertactin-Negative *Bordetella pertussis* Strains," *Clinical Infectious Diseases* 60:223, 2015.
8. Long, G., et al., "Acellular Pertussis Vaccination Facilitates *Bordetella parapertussis Infection,*" *Proceedings of the Royal Society of Biological Sciences* 10:1098, 2010.
9. Althouse, B., and Scarpino, S., "Asymptomatic Transmission and the Resurgence of *Bordetella pertussis,*" *BMC Medicine* 13:1186, 2015.
10. "Diphtheria," CDC, cdc.gov, and "Diphtheria, Reported Cases, 1980–2014, World Health Organization, who.int.
11. "Diphtheria Toxin," Wikipedia, en.wikipedia.org.

12. "Tetanus," CDC, cdc.gov.
13. "1900 United States Census," Wikipedia, en.wikipedia.org.
14. "Tetanus, Reported Cases, 1980–2014," WHO, who.int.
15. "Polio Vaccine Information Statement," CDC, cdc.gov.
16. "Ingredients: IPOL (IPV, Sanofi-Pasteur)," 2005, vaccines.ProCon.org.
17. Burnet, M., and White, D., *The Natural History of Infectious Disease*, Cambridge, 1972, p. 16.
18. Dubos, R., *Mirage of Health*, Harper, 1959, pp. 74–75.
19. Burnet and White, op. cit., p. 91 et seq.
20. Davis, B., et al., *Microbiology*, 2nd ed., Harper, 1973, p. 1290 et seq.
21. "Polio Outbreak Sparked by Vaccine, Experts Say," Associated Press, 2007, NBCNEWS.com.
22. Vashisht, N., et al., "Trends in Non-Polio Acute Flaccid Paralysis Incidence in India, 2000–2013," Supplement, *Pediatrics* 135: S16, 2015.
23. "Acute Flaccid Myelitis Surveillance, August 2014-July 2015," CDC, cdc.gov.
24. Ibid.
25. Greninger, A., et al., "A Novel Enterovirus D68 Strain Associated with Acute Flaccid Myelitis Cases in the USA (2012–2014): a Retrospective Cohort Study," *Lancet Infectious Diseases* 15:671, 2015.
26. Tao, Z., et al., "Non-Polio Enteroviruses from Acute Flaccid Paralysis Surveillance in Shandong Province, China, 1988–2014," nature.com/srep/, 2014.
27. Eddy, B., "Tumors Produced in Hamsters by SV40," *Federation Proceedings* 21:930, 1962.
28. Sweet, B., and Hillerman, M., "The Vacuolating Virus, SV40," *Proceedings of the Society for Experimental Biology* 105:420, 1960.
29. Institute of Medicine, "SV40 Contamination of Polio Vaccine and Cancer," *Immunization Safety Review* 4:21, 2002.
30. Cf., for example, Gurney, J., et al., "Trends in Cancer Incidence among Children in the US," *Cancer* 78:532, 1996.
31. Huang, H., "Identification of Human Brain Tumors of DNA Sequences Specific for SV40," *Brain Pathology* 9:33, 1999.
32. Matker, C., et al., The Biological Activities of SV40 and Possible Oncogenic Effects in Humans," *Monaldi Archives for Chest Disease* 53:193, 1998.
33. Rizzo, P., et al., "SV40 Is Present in Most US Human Mesotheliomas," Supplement, *Chest* 116:470, 1999.
34. Cf., for example, Brinster, R., et al., "Transgenic Mice Harboring SV40 Genes Develop Characteristic Brain Tumors," *Cell* 37:367, 1984; Matker, 1998,

op. cit.; and Cicala, C., et al., "SV40 Induces Mesotheliomas in Hamsters," *American Journal of Pathology* 142:1524, 1993.
35. Gazdar, A., et al., "SV40 and Human Tumours: Myth, Association, or Causality?" *National Reviews of Cancer* 2:957, 2002.
36. Horwin, M., "Simian Virus 40 (SV40): a Cancer-Causing Monkey Virus from FDA-Approved Vaccines," *Albany Law Journal of Science and Technology* 13:721, 2003.
37. "Ingredients: M-M-R II (MMR, Merck)," 2010, vaccines.ProCon.org.
38. Whitaker, J., and Poland, G., "Measles and Mumps Outbreaks in the United States: Think Globally, Vaccinate Locally" Editorial, *Vaccine* 32:4703, 2014.
39. Murti, M., et al., "Case of Vaccine-Associated Measles 5 Weeks Post-Immunization, British Columbia, Canada," *Eurosurveillance* 18:12, 2013.
40. Cf., for example, Edmondson, M., et al., "Mild Measles and Secondary Vaccine Failure during a Sustained Outbreak in a Highly-Vaccinated Population," *Journal of the AMA* 263:2457, 1990; Gustafson, T., et al., "Measles Outbreak in a Fully-Immunized Secondary School Population," *New England Journal of Medicine* 316:771, 1987; and Matson, D., et al., "Investigation of a Measles Outbreak in a Fully Vaccinated School Population," *Pediatric Infectious Disease Journal* 12:292, 1993.
41. Whitaker and Poland, *Vaccine,* 2014, op. cit.
42. Ibid.
43. Simpson, R., "Infectiousness of Communicable Diseases," *Lancet* 6734:549, 1952.
44. Dayan, G., et al., "Recent Resurgence of Mumps in the United States," *New England Journal of Medicine* 358:1581, 2008.
45. Ibid.
46. Barskey, A., et al., "Mumps Outbreaks in Orthodox Jewish Communities in the United States," *New England Journal of Medicine* 367:1704, 2012.
47. "Mumps Outbreak at Harvard Threatens Graduation," *NBC News,* April 28, 2016.
48. "Rubella," Wikipedia, en.wikipedia.org.

CHAPTER TWELVE

1. "Ingredients: Recombivax (Recombinant Hep B Vaccine, Merck)," 2011, vaccines.ProCon.org.
2. *Family Practice News,* August 1, 1992, p. 23.

3. Pevsner, G., Letter, *American Family Physician,* January 1994, p. 47.
4. "Ingredients: ActHIB (Hæmophilus B Conjugate Vaccine/Tetanus Toxoid Conjugate, Sanofi-Pasteur)," 2009, vaccines.ProCon.org.
5. Stratton K., et al., *Adverse Events Associated with Childhood Vaccines: Evidence Bearing on Causality,* Report of the Vaccine Safety Committee, Institute of Medicine, National Academies Press, 1994, Chapter 9, p. 236 et seq.
6. Vide supra, Chapter 9.
7. Bluestone, C., "Otitis Media in Children," *New England Journal of Medicine* 306:1399, 1982.
8. MacNeil, J., et al., "Current Epidemiology and Trends in Invasive HiB Disease, US, 1989–2008," *Clinical Infectious Diseases* 53:1230, 2011.
9. Cf., for example, Lipsitch, M., "Bacterial Vaccines and Serotype Replacement: Lessons from *Hæmophilus influenzæ* and Prospects for *Streptococcus pneumoniæ,*" *Emerging Infectious Diseases* 5, 1999, CDC, cdc.gov.
10. Ribeiro, G., et al., "Prevention of HiB Meningitis and Emergence of Serotype Replacement with Type A Strains after Introduction of HiB Immunization in Brazil," *Journal of Infectious Diseases* 187:109, 2003.
11. "Ingredients: Prevnar-13 (Pneumococcal Conjugate Vaccine, Wyeth)," 2012, vaccines.ProCon.org.
12. Simberkoff, M., et al., "Efficacy of Pneumococcal Vaccine in High-Risk Patients," *New England Journal of Medicine* 315:1318, 1986.
13. Whitney, C., et al., "Increasing Prevalence of Multidrug-Resistant *Streptococcus pneumoniæ* in the United States," *New England Journal of Medicine* 343:1917, 2000.
14. Eskola, J., "Efficacy of a Pneumococcal Conjugate Vaccine against Acute Otitis Media," *New England Journal of Medicine* 344:403, 2001.
15. *Family Practice News,* April 15, 2000, p. 1.
16. Cantekin, E., Letter, *New England Journal of Medicine* 344:1719, 2001.
17. Damoiseaux, R., Letter, ibid.
18. "Ingredients: Varivax (Varicella Live-Virus Vaccine, Merck)", 2011, vaccines. ProCon.org.
19. "Chickenpox," *AMA Encyclopedia of Medicine,* Random House, 1989, p. 262.
20. "Chickenpox," American Academy of Pediatrics brochure, 1996.
21. "The Vaccine for Chickenpox," *American Family Physician* 53:652, 1996, patient information handout.
22. Spingarn, R., and Benjamin, J., Letter, *New England Journal of Medicine* 338:683, 1998.

23. Shapiro, E., and LaRussa, P., "Vaccination for *Varicella*: Just Do It!" Editorial, *Journal of the AMA* 228:1529, 1997.
24. "Reported Cases and Deaths from Vaccine-Preventable Diseases, US, 1950–2011," CDC, cdc.gov., 2012.
25. Ibid.
26. Vide supra, Chapter 2.
27. Vide supra, Chapter 5.
28. Vide supra, Chapter 1.
29. "Ingredients: RotaTeq (Rotavirus, Live-Virus Vaccine, Merck, Oral, Pentavalent)," 2011, vaccines.ProCon.org.
30. "Rotavirus Vaccine Information Statement," CDC, cdc.gov., 2015.
31. Tucker, A., et al., "Cost-Effectiveness Analysis of a Rotavirus Immunization Program for the United States," *Journal of the AMA* 279:1371, 1998.
32. Ibid.
33. Keusch, G., and Cash, R., "A Vaccine against Rotavirus: When Is Too Much Too Much?" Editorial, *New England Journal of Medicine* 337:1228, 1997.
34. Vide supra, Chapters 5, 8.
35. Murphy, T., et al., "Intussusception among Infants Given an Oral Rotavirus Vaccine," *New England Journal of Medicine* 344:564, 2001.
36. Ibid.
37. Offit, P., "Addressing Parents' Concerns: Do Multiple Vaccines Overwhelm or Weaken the Infant's Immune System?" *Pediatrics* 109:124, 2002.
38. Handley, J., "Dr. Paul Offit: Fox in the Henhouse, the ACIP Years (1998–2003)," ageofautism.com, 2009.
39. "Inactivated or Recombinant Influenza Vaccine: Information Statement," CDC, cdc.gov., 2015.
40. "Ingredients: Fluarix (Quadrivalent Influenza Vaccine, GlaxoSmithKline)," 2013, vaccines.ProCon.org.
41. For this and the following details of this history, I am largely indebted to Drs. Eric Biondi and Andrew Aligne, whose splendid article, "Flu Vaccine for All: a Critical Look at the Evidence," appeared on *Medscape Pediatrics,* December 21, 2015, www.medscape.com/pediatrics.
42. Francis, T., et al., "Experience with Vaccination against Influenza in the Spring of 1947," *American Journal of Public Health* 37:1017, 1947.
43. Henderson, D., et al., "Public Health and Medical Responses to the 1957–58 Influenza Pandemic," *Biosecurity and Bioterrorism* 7:265, 2009.
44. Langmuir, A., et al., "The Epidemiological Basis for the Control of Influenza," *American Journal of Public Health* 54:563, 1964.

45. Schoenbaum, S., et al., "Studies with Inactivated Influenza Vaccines: Efficacy," *Bulletin of the World Health Organization* 41:531, 1969.
46. Sencer, D., and Millar, J., "Reflections on the 1976 Swine Flu Vaccination Program," *Emerging Infectious Diseases:* 12:29, 2006.
47. Dull, H., and Bryan, J., "Assuring the Benefits of Immunization in the Future: Research in the Public Interest," *Bulletin of the World Health Organization,* Supplement 2, 55:117, 1977.
48. Vide supra, Chapter 3.
49. Gross, P., et al., "The Efficacy of Influenza Vaccine in Elderly Persons: a Meta-analysis and Review of the Literature," *Annals of Internal Medicine* 123:518, 1995.
50. Bridges C., et al., "Effectiveness and Cost-Benefit of Influenza Vaccination of Healthy Working Adults: a Randomized, Controlled Trial," *Journal of the AMA* 284:1655, 2000.
51. "Recommendations for Influenza Immunization in Children," American Academy of Pediatrics Committee on Infectious Diseases, *Pediatrics* 113:1441, 2004.
52. "Influenza Immunization for All Health Care Personnel: Keep It Mandatory," American Academy of Pediatrics Committee on Infectious Diseases, *Pediatrics* 136:809, 2015.
53. Nichol, K., et al., "The Effectiveness of Vaccination against Influenza in Healthy Working Adults," *New England Journal of Medicine* 333:889, 1995.
54. "Flu Vaccine Safety and Pregnancy," CDC, cdc.gov., 2014.
55. Matanoski, V., "Adjudicated Settlements, 3rd Quarter 2013," Department of Justice, hrsa.gov.
56. Ibid. I have omitted a few of the awards for reactions to a combination of vaccines when they included the influenza.
57. "Fluarix," *Physicians' Desk Reference,* 70th ed., 2016, p. 956.
58. Vide supra, Chapter 8.

CHAPTER THIRTEEN

1. "Meningococcal Disease," CDC, cdc.gov.
2. Ibid.
3. "Meningococcal Disease," *The History of Vaccines,* Philadelphia College of Physicians, historyofvaccines.org.
4. "Meningococcal State Mandates for Elementary and Secondary Schools," Immunization Action Coalition, immunize.org.

5. "Ingredients: Meningococcal Vaccines MCV4-Menactra (Sanofi-Pasteur), MenHibrix (GSK), Menveo (Novartis), and Menoimmune (Sanofi-Pasteur), vaccines.ProCon.org.
6. "The Crap in Vaccines: Meningococcal Vaccines Produced in *E. Coli*," WordPress.com, February 5, 2016.
7. Robert F. Kennedy, Jr., "Doing the Math on Meningitis Vaccinations," *Boulder Daily Camera*, June 9, 2015.
8. "Hepatitis A," CDC, cdc.gov.
9. "Hepatitis A Fact Sheet," World Health Organization, who.int.
10. "Hepatitis A State Mandates for Daycare and K-12," Immunization Action Coalition, immunize.org.
11. "Hepatitis A," CDC, op. cit.
12. "Havrix" (GSK) and "Vaqta" (Merck), *Physicians' Desk Reference*, 70th ed., 2016, pp. 964–5, 1583.
13. "Ingredients: Havrix (Hep A Vaccine, GSK) and Vaqta (Hep A Vaccine, Merck)," vaccines.ProCon.org.
14. "Cervical Cancer," National Cancer Institute, NIH, cancer.gov.
15. Ibid.
16. Ibid.
17. Castellsagué, X., et al., "Risk of Newly-Detected Infections and Cervical Abnormalities in Women Seropositive for Naturally-Acquired HPV-16 and HPV-18 Antibodies," *Journal of Infectious Diseases* 10:1093, online version March 8, 2014.
18. "Cervical Cancer Screening," National Cancer Institute, NIH, cancer.gov.
19. "Cervical Cancer," National Cancer Institute, op. cit.
20. "Ingredients: HPV Recombinant Vaccines Cervarix (bivalent, GSK) and Gardasil (quadrivalent, Merck), vaccines.ProCon.org.
21. Slade, B., et al., "Postlicensure Safety Surveillance for Quadrivalent HPV Recombinant Vaccine," *Journal of the AMA* 302:750, 2009.
22. As we saw in chapter 3, the safety trials listed in the package insert indicate that 5088 women and girls received Gardasil, 3,470 received the aluminum adjuvant alone, and only 320 received saline, whereas for the serious adverse reactions the two so-called "placebo control" groups were combined, so that the small number of reactions to the saline were hidden in the much larger total for the aluminum group.
23. Tomljenovic, L., and Shaw, C., "HPV Vaccine Policy and Evidence-Based Medicine: Are They at Odds?" *Annals of Medicine* Online, Informa UK, Ltd., p. 1, informahealthcare.com, 2011.

24. "Tens of Thousands of Teen Girls Suffer Serious Illnesses after HPV Cervical Cancer Jab," London *Daily Express,* January 1, 2015.
25. "Gardasil," *Physicians' Desk Reference,* 70th ed., 2016, pp. 1336–37.
26. Brinth, L., et al., "Orthostatic Intolerance and Postural Tachycardia Syndrome as Suspected Adverse Effects of Vaccination against HPV," *Vaccine* 33:2602, 2015.
27. Colafrancesco, S., et al., "HPV Vaccine and Primary Ovarian Failure: Another Facet of the Autoimmune (Inflammatory) Syndrome Induced by Adjuvants (ASIA)," *American Journal of Reproductive Immunology* 70:309, 2013.
28. Field, S., "New Concerns about the HPV Vaccine," American College of Pediatricians, acpeds.org, January 2016.
29. "Two ALS Cases May Be Linked to Gardasil," *WebMD* News Archive, October 16, 2009.
30. Cf., for example, Gomez v. Secretary of HHS, VICP claim #15-0160V, in which a 14-year-old boy died in his sleep the day after receiving his second HPV shot; Dave Hodges, "The Murdering of Our Daughters," *The Common Sense Show,* September 17, 2013, in which the deaths of eight adolescent girls are detailed; "6248 Permanent Injuries and 144 Deaths Following Gardasil: Coincidence or Scandal?" *Health Impact News,* December 10, 2013, culled from 31,741 VAERS reports, as of November 2013; and "Girl with Sore Throat Gets HPV Vaccine, Dies Hours Later," *Fox 4 Newsroom,* August 11, 2014.
31. Lee, S., "Detection of HPV L.1 Gene DNA Fragments in Postmortem Blood and Spleen after Gardasil Vaccination: a Case Report," *Advances in Bioscience and Biotechnology* 3:1214, 2012.
32. Gilkey, M., et al., "Quality of Physician Communication about HPV Vaccine: a National Survey," *Cancer Epidemiology, Biomarkers, and Prevention* 24:1673, 2015.
33. Interview with Sharyl Attkisson, *CBS News,* August 19, 2009.
34. Interview with *Principes de Santé,* April 2014, cited in *Health Impact News,* healthimpactnews.com, October 29, 2014.
35. *Tokyo Times,* July 1, 2014.
36. Ibid.
37. "Gardasil: Criminal Complaint Filed in Spain," Sanevax, Inc., sanevax.org., August 2, 2014.
38. "Gardasil Firestorm in Denmark," Sanevax, Inc., sanevax.org, June 21, 2015.
39. Ibid.
40. Ibid.

41. London *Daily Mail,* January 13, 2015.
42. "HPV Controversy in Colombia Continues," Sanevax, Inc., sanevax.org, April 11, 2015.
43. "Independent Medical Researchers Agree with Parents," *Health Impact News,* heathimpactnews.com, April 13, 2015.
44. Tomljenovic and Shaw, "Too Fast or Not Too Fast; FDA Approval of Merck's HPV Vaccine Gardasil," *Journal of Law, Medicine, and Ethics* 40:673, 2012.
45. Cf., for example, Gostin, L., "Mandatory HPV Vaccination and Political Debate," *Journal of the AMA* 306:1699, 2011: "If mandatory vaccination proves unsuccessful, states should seriously consider compulsory vaccination laws without generous exemptions."
46. "Fast Track, Accelerated Approval, and Priority Review," FDA, fda.gov, September 2012, and Harper, D., et al., "Cervical Cancer Incidence Can Increase Despite HPV Vaccination," *Lancet Infectious Diseases* 10:594, 2010.
47. Ostor, A., "Natural History of Cervical Intraepithelial Neoplasia: a Critical Review," *International Journal of Gynecological Pathology* 12:186, 1993.
48. Harper, D., and Williams, K., "Prophylactic HPV Vaccines: Current Knowledge of Impact on Gynecological Premalignancy," *Discovery Medicine* 10:7, 2010.
49. "Summary of Adverse Reactions Following Vaccination with Gardasil in the U. S. Reported to VAERS, June 2006-September 2012," Table 1, Tomljenovic and Shaw, 2012, op. cit., tabulated from VAERS Internet Database, CDC, wonder.cdc.gov/vaers, September 2012.
50. Ibid., Table 2, "Age-Adjusted Rate of Adverse Reactions to Gardasil and Other Vaccines," tabulated from VAERS Internet Database, September 2012, op. cit.
51. Exley, C., "Aluminum-Based Adjuvants Should not Be Used as Placebos in Clinical Trials," *Vaccine* 29:2989, 2011, and Shoenfeld, Y., and Agmon-Levin, N., "ASIA Syndrome," *Journal of Autoimmunity* 36:4, 2011.
52. Tomljenovic and Shaw, 2011, op. cit.
53. "Medicines in Development: Vaccines," Press Release, PhRMA, phrma.org, September 11, 2013.
54. Ibid.
55. Zimmer, C., "Protection Without a Vaccine," *New York Times,* March 9, 2015.
56. Ibid.
57. McDonnell, W., and Askari, F., "The Emerging role of DNA Vaccines," *Medscape,* July 30, 2008.
58. Ibid.

59. Zimmer, 2015, op. cit.
60. Shanahan, C., "Humans as GMO's? New Vaccine Technology Alters Our DNA," *Dr. Cate,* drcate.com, December 16, 2009.

CHAPTER FOURTEEN

1. World Medical Association, *Ethical Principles for Medical Research Involving Human Subjects,* Helsinki, 1964, amended 2008, ¶32, p. 5, and *The Nuremberg Code,* 1947, Wikipedia, ¶1.
2. Mendelsohn, R., "The Devil's Priests," in *Confessions of a Medical Heretic,* Contemporary Books, 1979.
3. Dubos, R., *Mirage of Health,* Harper, 1959, p. 157.
4. "Inoculations Put Aspin in the Hospital," *Boston Globe,* February 23, 1993, p. 1.
5. Attkisson, S., "What the News Isn't Saying About Vaccine-Autism Studies," sharylattkisson.com, April 25, 2015.
6. Vide supra, Chapter 4, StopMandatoryVaccination.com.
7. In addition to Stop Mandatory Vaccination, among the many other groups involved were the National Vaccine Information Center, Parental Rights.org, the Pacific Justice Committee, National Health Freedom Action, the Eagle Forum of California, California Nurses for Ethical Solutions, the Libertarian Party of Sacramento County, the Weston Price Foundation, the California ProLife Council, and the Canary Party, all members of the California Coalition for Vaccine Choice.
8. Revolt.Revoke.Restore, revoltrevokerestore.com, March 1, 2016.
9. Posfe-Barbe, K., et al., "How Do Physicians Immunize Their Own Children?" *Pediatrics* 116:623, 2005.
10. Gust, D., et al., "Physicians Who Do and Do Not Recommend Children Get All Vaccinations," *Journal of Health Communication* 13:573, 2008.
11. Clark, S., et al., "Influenza Vaccination Attitudes and Practices among US Registered Nurses," *American Journal of Infection Control* 37:551, 2009.
12. "Nurses Taking a Stand Against Forced Flu Vaccines," *Health Impact News,* healthimpactnews.com, January 4, 2014.
13. "Boston Nurses Speak Out Against Mandatory Flu Shots," *Health Impact News,* healthimpctnews.com, October 20, 2014.
14. "Recommended Immunization Schedule for Persons Age 0–18 Years," ACIP, cdc.gov/vaccines/acip, 2016.

15. Eickhoff, T., "Adult Immunizations: How Are We Doing?" *Hospital Practice,* November 15, 1996, p. 107.
16. "Recommended Adult Immunization Schedule," ACIP, cdc.gov/vaccines/acip, 2016.
17. Peter, G., "Childhood Immunizations," *New England Journal of Medicine* 327:1794, 1992.
18. Cf. "State Mandates on Immunization," Immunization Action Coalition, immunize.org, and "School Vaccination Requirements," CDC, cdc.gov.
19. "States with Religious and Philosophical Exemptions from School Immunization Requirements," National Conference of State legislatures, or NCSL, ncsl.org.
20. Vide supra, Chapter 3.
21. Vide supra, Chapter 6.
22. Ibid.
23. Ibid.
24. "Former CDC Director Sells 38,368 Shares of Merck Stock for $2.3 million," *Health Impact News,* healthimpactnews.com, May 25, 2015: "Julie Gerberding was in charge of the CDC from 2002–09, the years when the FDA approved Merck's Gardasil vaccine. Soon after she took over the CDC, she overhauled the agency's organizational structure, and many of the senior scientists left. Some claim that most replacements she appointed had ties to the vaccine industry. Dr. Gerberding resigned from the CDC in 2009, and took over as president of Merck's Vaccine division, a $5 billion a year operation, and supplier of the largest number of CDC-recommended vaccines. It was reported earlier that Gerberding, now executive vice president of Merck, sold 38,368 shares for $2,340,064. She still holds 31,985 shares, valued at $2 million."
25. "Former Merck Rep Says Vaccination Is for Profit, Not Public Health," StopMandatoryVaccination.com, July 26, 2015: "Brandy Vaughan, a former sales rep for Merck, has found from her own research that vaccines contain known toxins that can cause neurological damage, and that their safety studies lack the same standards as are required for other drugs. She has decided against vaccinating her own children, saying that it's like playing Russian roulette, and that mandatory vaccination is simply a vehicle for generating massive profits."
26. Gwen Olsen, *Confessions of an Ex Drug Pusher*, iUniverse, 2009.
27. "Drug Companies Donated Millions to California Lawmakers Before Vaccine Debate," *Sacramento Bee,* June 18, 2015, sacbee.com: "Critics of SB

277 accuse the measure's supporters in the Legislature of doing the bidding of donors who make vaccines and other pharmaceuticals. Drug companies and trade groups did give more than $2 million to current members of the Legislature in 2013–2014, records show. The top recipient is Senator Richard Pan, a Sacramento Democrat and doctor who is carrying the vaccine bill; he got more than $95,000. The industry donated more than $500,000 to outside campaign spending groups that helped elect some current members, and spent nearly $3 million during the 2013–2014 legislative session lobbying the Legislature, the governor, the state pharmacists' board and other agencies, according to state filings."

28. Angell, M., "Big Pharma, Bad Medicine," *Boston Review,* May 1, 2010.
29. Angell, source unknown, cited in "Pertinent Quotes from Marcia Angell, MD," *PPJ Gazette,* February 2015, compiled by Gary Kohls, MD.
30. Angell, "Health: the Right Diagnosis and the Wrong Treatment," *New York Review of Books,* April 23, 2015, p. 44.
31. Ibid., p. 47.

SUGGESTIONS FOR FURTHER READING

GENERAL

I found the following books especially helpful for an overview of the subject from various points of view:

Louise Habakus, MA, and Mary Holland, JD, eds., *Vaccine Epidemic,* Skyhorse, 2011. Contains articles by a diverse group of experts on a wide array of scientific, clinical, and legal topics bearing on vaccination as a human rights issue. Excellent.

Suzanne Humphries, MD, and Roman Bystrianyk, *Dissolving Illusions,* 2013, www.dissolvingillusions.com. Provides valuable historical and clinical perspective on both vaccination in general and the individual vaccines in particular.

Sherri Tenpenny, DO, *Saying No to Vaccines: a Resource Guide for All Ages,* Tenpenny Publishing, 2008. A comprehensive view of the entire subject, from the point of view of an experienced clinician. Authoritative, well researched, and highly recommended.

Paul Offit, MD, *Vaccinated: One Man's Quest to Defeat the World's Deadliest Diseases,* HarperCollins, 2007. A spirited defense of our current vaccine policy by one of its leading advocates, a long-time member of the official CDC Advisory Committee on Immunization Practices, as well as the principal developer of Merck's RotaTeq vaccine.

Harris L. Coulter, PhD, and Barbara Loe Fisher, *DPT: a Shot in the Dark,* Harcourt Brace Jovanovich, 1985. A ground-breaking book that helped launch the national movement for informed consent, vaccination choice, and safer vaccines, based on the personal histories of dozens of children who suffered major brain damage after their DPT vaccinations.

Neil Z. Miller, *Review of Critical Vaccine Studies,* New Atlantean Press, 2016. Well-researched, comprehensive, up-to-date review of the scientific and clinical literature documenting adverse effects of vaccinations. Over 400 peer-reviewed studies are summarized. Invaluable.

Yehuda Shoenfeld, PhD, Nancy Agmon-Levin, PhD, and Lucija Tomljenovic, PhD, eds., *Vaccines and Autoimmunity,* WILEY Blackwell, 2015. A compendium of pioneering, scholarly contributions by many prominent scientists on the autoimmune mechanisms involved in the vaccination process, and the diverse autoimmune diseases exhibited by vaccinated patients. Essential reading.

CHAPTER ONE

Harold Buttram, MD, "Current Childhood Vaccination Programs: an Overview," *Medical Veritas,* 2008.

CHAPTER TWO

Herbert Ratner, MD, et al., "The Present State of Polio Vaccines," *Illinois Medical Journal* 118:84 and 118:160, 1969.

Barbara Loe Fisher, *The Emerging Risks of Live-Virus and Virus-Vectored Vaccines: Vaccine-Strain Virus Infection, Shedding, and Transmission*, National Vaccine Information Center, www.NVIC.org, 2014.

James Cherry, MD, "The New Epidemiology of Measles and Rubella," *Hospital Practice,* July 1980.

CHAPTER THREE

Dr. Colleen Boyle, in reply to questioning by Rep. Bill Posey (R-FL), House Oversight and Government Reform Committee, November 29, 2012.

"ActHiB," Package Insert, Sanofi-Pasteur, 2009.

"Gardasil," Package Insert, Merck, 2015.

Interview with Dr. Peter Rost, in Gardasil documentary, *One More Girl,* www.collective-evolution.com, July 7, 2015.

World Medical Association, *Ethical Principles for Medical Research Involving Human Subjects,* Helsinki, 1964, amended 2008, 32, p. 5.

The Nuremberg Code, 1947, Wikipedia, 1.

Marcia Angell, MD, "Drug Companies and Doctors: a Story of Corruption," *New York Review of Books,* January 15, 2009.

Angell, "Big Pharma, Bad Medicine," *Boston Review,* May 1, 2010.

CHAPTER FOUR

Robert Mendelsohn, MD, *How to Raise a Healthy Child . . . in Spite of Your Doctor,* Contemporary Books, 1984.

Larry Cook, "Parents Share Why They'll Never Vaccinate Again," www.StopMandatoryVaccination.com.

Richard Moskowitz, MD, "Hidden in Plain Sight: the Role of Vaccines in Chronic Disease," *American Journal of Homeopathic Medicine* 98:15, Spring 2005.

Moskowitz, "The Case against Immunizations," *Journal of the American Institute of Homeopathy* 76:7, 1983.

Moskowitz, "Vaccination: a Sacrament of Modern Medicine," *Journal of the American Institute of Homeopathy* 84:96, December 1991.

Moskowitz, "Childhood Ear Infections," *Journal of the American Institute of Homeopathy* 87:137, Autumn 1994.

Moskowitz, "Hidden in Plain Sight: Vaccines as a Major Risk Factor for Chronic Disease," *American Journal of Homeopathic Medicine* 106:107, Autumn 2013.

CHAPTER FIVE

Andrew Wakefield, MD, et al., "Measles Vaccine: a Risk Factor for Inflammatory Bowel Disease?" *Lancet* 345:1071, 1995.

Wakefield, et al., "Ileal-Lymphoid Hyperplasia, Nonspecific Colitis, and Pervasive Developmental Disorder in Children," *Lancet* 351:637, 1998.

Lucija Tomljenovic, PhD, and Christopher Shaw, PhD, "Answers to Common Misconceptions Regarding the Toxicity of Aluminum Adjuvants in Vaccines," *Vaccines and Autoimmunity,* op. cit., Chapter 4.

Shaw, et al., "Aluminum Hydroxide Injections Lead to Motor Deficits and Motor Neuron Degeneration," *Journal of Inorganic Biochemistry* 103:1555, 2009.

Tomljenovic, "Aluminum and Alzheimer's Disease: after a Century of Controversy, Is There a Plausible Link?" *Journal of Alzheimer's Disease* 23:567, 2011.

Stephanie Seneff, PhD, "Empirical Data Confirm Autism Symptoms Related to Aluminum and Acetaminophen Exposure," *Entropy* 14:2227, 2012.

Drs. Shoenfeld and Agmon-Levin, "ASIA: Autoimmune/Inflammatory Syndrome Induced by Adjuvants," *Journal of Autoimmunity* 36:4, 2011.

Paul Offit, MD, et al., "Addressing Parents' Concerns: Do Vaccines Contain Harmful Preservatives, Adjuvants, Additives, or Residuals?" *Pediatrics* 112:1394, 2003.

CHAPTER SIX

Gordon Stewart, MD, "Vaccination against Whooping-Cough: Efficacy vs. Risks," *Lancet* 309:234, 1977.

"Vaccine Side Effects, Adverse Reactions, Contraindications & Precautions," Advisory Committee on Immunization Practices, *Morbidity and Mortality Weekly Report* 45:22, 1996.

Leo Kanner, MD, "Autistic Disturbances of Affective Contact," *Nervous Child* 2:217, 1943.

Dr. Wakefield, "Autism and Childhood Vaccines," Congressional Testimony, C-Span, April 6, 2000.

Wakefield, "MMR, Enterocolitis, and Autism," Lecture, NVIC International Conference, Washington, DC, 2002.

Mary Megson, MD, "Genetics, Vaccine Injury, and Getting Well," Lecture, NVIC International Conference, op. cit.

Written Statement of William Thompson, PhD, submitted to Rep. William Posey (R-FL), read *verbatim* in Congress, excerpted by Sharyl Attkisson, CBS News, July 29, 2015.

Robert F. Kennedy Jr. "Central Figure in CDC Vaccine Cover-up Absconds with $2 million," *Huffington Post,* May 11, 2010.

RFK Jr., ed., *Thimerosal: Let the Science Speak,* Skyhorse, 2014.

CHAPTER SEVEN

CDC, "About SUID and SIDS," www.cdc.gov.

Dr. Cherry, et al., "Report of Task Force on Pertussis and Pertussis Immunization," Supplement, *Pediatrics* 81:939, 1988.

Viera Scheibner, PhD, *Vaccination: a Medical Assault on the Immune System,* New Atlantean Press, 1993.

"Personal Stories of Vaccine Injury and Death," www.thinktwice.com, Think Twice Global Vaccine Institute.

Dr. Offit, et al., "Addressing Parents' Concerns: Do Multiple Vaccines Overwhelm or Weaken the Infant's Immune System?" *Pediatrics* 109:124, 2002.

Barbara Loe Fisher, "In Memoriam: Infant Death and Vaccination," *The Vaccine Reaction,* NVIC, May 25, 2011.

CHAPTER EIGHT

Mary Holland, JD, "Unanswered Questions from the Vaccine Injury Compensation Program: a Review of Uncompensated Cases of Vaccine-Induced Brain Injury," *Pace Environmental Law Review* 28:480, March 28, 2011.

"Vaccine Safety Post-Marketing Surveillance: the Vaccine Adverse Event Reporting System," CDC, www.vaers.hhs.gov, 2004.

CDC, "Table of Reportable Events Following Vaccination," www.cdc.gov/vaccines, 2008.

"Vaccine Injury Table," Health Resources and Services Administration, www.hrsa.gov, Department of Health and Human Services, June 23, 2015.

Wayne Rohde, *The Vaccine Court,* Skyhorse, 2014

Barbara Loe Fisher, "Vaccine Injury Compensation: Government's Broken Social Contract with Parents," *The Vaccine Reaction,* November 2, 2015, www.nvic.org.

CHAPTER NINE

Dan Olmsted, "The Amish All Over Again," *Age of Autism,* May 12, 2012, www.ageofautism.com.

Sharyl Attkisson, "Where Are the Autistic Amish?" www.sharylattkisson.com, July 20, 2014.

Sue Claridge, "Unvaccinated Children Are Healthier," *Investigate before You Vaccinate,* www.vaccineinjury.info, 2005.

CHAPTER TEN

Dr. Tomljenovic, "Aluminum and Alzheimer's Disease," *Journal of Alzheimer's Disease* 23:567, 2011.

Christopher Exley, PhD, "Aluminium and Medicine," in *Molecular and Supramolecular Bio-Inorganic Chemistry,* Nova Biomedical Books, 2009.

Romain Gherardi, MD, et al., "Central Nervous System Disease in Patients with Macrophagic Myofascitis," *Brain* 124:974, 2001.

Gherardi, "Lessons from Macrophagic Myofasciitis: Towards Definition of a Vaccine Adjuvant-Related Syndrome," *Revue Neurologique* (Paris) 159:162, 2003.

Exley, et al., "Elevated Urinary Excretion of Aluminium and Iron in Multiple Sclerosis," *Multiple Sclerosis* 12:533, 2006.

Russell Blaylock, MD, et al., "Immune Glutamatergic Dysfunction as a Central Mechanism of Autism-Spectrum Disorders," *Current Medicinal Chemistry* 16:157, 2009.

Tomljenovic and Shaw, "Aluminum Vaccine Adjuvants: Are They Safe?" *Current Medicinal Chemistry* 18:2630, 2011.

Larry Palevsky, MD, "Aluminum and Vaccine Ingredients: What Do We Know? What Don't We Know?" *International Medical Council on Vaccination*, 2009.

CHAPTER ELEVEN

Dr. Cherry, et al., "Report of Task Force on Pertussis and Pertussis Immunization," Supplement, *Pediatrics* 81:939, 1988.

Sir Macfarlane Burnet, PhD, *The Natural History of Infectious Disease*, Cambridge, 1972.

René Dubos, PhD, *Mirage of Health*, Harper, 1959.

Bernice Eddy, PhD, "Tumors Produced in Hamsters by SV40," *Federation Proceedings* 21:930, 1962.

"Mumps Outbreak at Harvard Threatens Graduation," *NBC News*, April 28, 2016.

"Vaccine Ingredients," www.ProCon.org.

CHAPTER TWELVE

Charles Bluestone, MD, "Otitis Media in Children," *New England Journal of Medicine* 306:1399, 1982.

Eric Biondi, MD, and Andrew Aligne, MD, "Flu Vaccine for All: a Critical Look at the Evidence," *Medscape Pediatrics*, www.medscape.com/pediatrics, Dec 21, 2015.

CHAPTER THIRTEEN

RFK Jr., "Doing the Math on Meningitis Vaccinations," *Boulder Daily Camera*, June 9, 2015.

Tomljenovic and Shaw, "HPV Vaccine Policy and Evidence-Based Medicine: Are They at Odds?" *Annals of Medicine* Online, www.informahealthcare.com, 2011.

Tomljenovic and Shaw, "Too Fast or Not Too Fast; FDA Approval of Merck's HPV Vaccine Gardasil," *Journal of Law, Medicine, and Ethics* 40:673, 2012.

Drs. McDonnell and Askari, "The Emerging role of DNA Vaccines," *Medscape,* July 30, 2008.

CHAPTER FOURTEEN

"Recommended Immunization Schedule for Persons Age 0–18 Years," ACIP, www.cdc.gov/vaccines/acip, 2016.

"Recommended Adult Immunization Schedule," ACIP, www.cdc.gov/vaccines/acip, 2016.

Georges Peter, MD, "Childhood Immunizations," *New England Journal of Medicine* 327:1794, 1992.

Dr. Angell, "Big Pharma, Bad Medicine," *Boston Review,* May 1, 2010.

Angell, "Health: the Right Diagnosis and the Wrong Treatment," *New York Review of Books,* April 23, 2015.

ACKNOWLEDGMENTS

First of all, I want to thank Louis Conte and Tony Lyons at Skyhorse for their interest in the book, and my Skyhorse editors for helping me work it through to the point where we were all satisfied with it.

Secondly, I'm deeply grateful to Mary Holland, the legal scholar and human rights activist whose many valuable suggestions were based on careful study of the text, and to Drs. Janet Levatin, Michelle Dossett, Ron Whitmont, and Karl Robinson, physician-colleagues who reviewed selected chapters and provided helpful comments.

Third, I want to pay tribute to the many practicing physicians, both living and deceased, whose investigations and thoughts about vaccines have aided and inspired my own, including but by no means limited to Drs. Robert Mendelsohn, Mayer Eisenstein, Harold Buttram, Gordon Stewart, Philip Incao, Larry Palevsky, Toni Bark, Janet Levatin, Kris Gaublomme, Tinus Smits, Sherri Tenpenny, Suzanne Humphries, Marcia Angell, and of course Andrew Wakefield, whose findings that autism is an autoimmune condition with measles antibodies and lesions of inflammatory bowel disease have opened up a vast new field of study.

Fourth, I'm indebted to a number of research scientists whose experimental work has directly influenced my own, especially Viera Scheibner, Yehuda Shoenfeld, Lucia Tomljenovic, Chris Shaw, Chris Exley, Gary Goldman, Tetyana Obukhanych, and Stephanie Seneff. The complete list is of course much longer.

Fifth, I want to acknowledge several dedicated investigative journalists, especially Neil Miller who has been challenging the official whitewash of vaccines for decades, and whose excellent resource book, *Review of Critical Vaccine Studies*, reliably directed me to pertinent research; and Sharyl Attkisson, Ben Swann, Dan

Olmsted, Del Bigtree, and Robert F. Kennedy Jr. who have had the courage to see through the propaganda and follow the real stories beyond the headlines.

Sixth, I want to express my appreciation for all of the activists who have been working tirelessly on behalf of the vaccine-injured, including their own children in many cases, often without pay, and advocating for safer vaccines, parental choice, and compensation of victims. Although the actual number is much larger, I will single out a few whose work I happen to be familiar with, namely, Greg Wyatt, Heather Leann, Brandy Vaughan, Mark Blaxill, Mary Aspinwall, and Marcella Piper-Terry; Larry Cook, of Stop Mandatory Vaccination; Terri Aranga, of AutismOne; Attorney Alan Phillips, representing the vaccine-injured; Mary Holland, JD, of New York University Law School; Louise Kuo Habakus of the Center for Personal Rights in New York; and above all Barbara Loe Fisher, whose record of dedicated advocacy spans thirty-five years, and Marco Càceres and the staff of the National Vaccine Information Center, her brainchild and ongoing life's work.

But the ultimate inspiration for this book are the thousands upon thousands of vaccine-injured children and adults, who have endured and must continue to endure various forms of brain damage, death, autoimmune diseases of every description, and injuries and illnesses of infinite variety, the vast majority of them unrecognized, written off as preexisting tendency or "coincidence," or simply denied altogether, as well as their parents, relatives, and friends, who know the truth of what really happened, and cannot rest until it is acknowledged, redeemed, or at least somehow atoned for.

ABOUT THE AUTHOR

Richard Moskowitz is a family physician specializing in homeopathic medicine. He received his BA from Harvard in 1959, Phi Beta Kappa, and his MD from New York University in 1963. After a Graduate Fellowship in Philosophy at the University of Colorado, he served a rotating internship at St. Anthony's Hospital in Denver from 1966 to 1967, and has been practicing family medicine ever since.

Attending over six hundred home births between 1969 and 1982, he also studied Japanese acupuncture with Sensei Masahilo Nakazono in Santa Fe, and classical homeopathy with Prof. George Vithoulkas in Athens, Dr. Rajan Sankaran and his school in Mumbai, and many other teachers. Homeopathic medicine has been his principal treatment modality since 1974.

In addition to teaching and lecturing, he has written four other books, *Homeopathic Medicines for Pregnancy and Childbirth* (1991); *Resonance: the Homeopathic Point of View* (2001); *Plain Doctoring: Selected Writings, 1983–2013* (2014); and *More Doctoring: Selected Writings, Vol. 2, 1977–2014* (2015), as well as numerous articles on homeopathy and the philosophy of medicine, including "Homeopathic Reasoning," "Why I Became a Homeopath," "Plain Doctoring," "Some Thoughts on the Malpractice Crisis," "Hidden in Plain Sight: the Rôle of Vaccines in Chronic Disease," "Diagnosis," and "For Homeopathy: a Practicing Physician's Perspective."

He is seventy-eight, married with two children and three grandchildren, and lives and practices in the Boston area.

INDEX